Endorsements

Step by mindful step, Cheryl confronts cancer with a peaceful mind. A great teaching for us all.
— JOSEPH GOLDSTEIN, author
Mindfulness: A Practical Guide to Awakening

This is a beautiful offering to fellow travelers—full of wisdom, hope, and deep compassion. By surrendering to the reality of cancer, Cheryl opens her heart to the fullness of this precious life.
— TARA BRACH, Ph.D. and author
Radical Acceptance and *True Refuge*

Mindfulness can allow you to stride through impossible situations like a colossus, in contact with a form of happiness that is independent of conditions. Sooner or later, every human being will have to face something seemingly unfaceable. Cheryl shows you how to do that. So there are two reasons you should read this book: information and inspiration.
— SHINZEN YOUNG, author
The Science of Enlightenment

Reading this book is like chatting and laughing with good friend, while also exploring a profound confrontation with life and death. In funny, heartfelt, so-down-to-earth ways, Cheryl Wilfong offers many useful perspectives and practices for anyone dealing with anything—and especially for people coping with the really big stuff.

— RICK HANSON, Ph.D. and author
Buddha's Brain: The Practical Neuroscience of Happiness, Love, and Wisdom

In *Breast Cancer Meets Mindfulness* Cheryl Wilfong takes the reader on her intimate journey with breast cancer. Steeped in wisdom and yet down-to-earth, the book helps us see the deep lessons and gifts hidden in wisely facing our mortality. A valuable offering.

— JAMES BARAZ, author
Awakening Joy: 10 Steps to Happiness and
co-founding teacher, Spirit Rock Meditation Center, Woodacre, CA

Intimate and unflinching, this account shows how our spiritual practice can guide us in meeting the grand emergency of cancer with kindness and compassion.

— SANDY BOUCHER, author
Hidden Spring: A Buddhist Woman Confronts Cancer

In this moving and insightful book, Cheryl shows how meditation and the Buddha's teaching became her refuge in the midst of the uncertainty and anxiety of a cancer diagnosis and treatment. Anyone can walk Cheryl's path and this makes the book universal. I highly recommend it.

—TONI BERNHARD, author

How to Be Sick: A Buddhist-Inspired Guide for the Chronically Ill and Their Caregivers
How to Wake Up: A Buddhist-Inspired Guide for Navigating Joy and Sorrow
How to Live Well with Chronic Pain and Illness: A Mindful Guide

In this warm and personal book Cheryl shares with us the power of heart cultivation. Her Dhamma practice enables her to embrace a diagnosis that is often marked by overwhelming fear and aversion. With her spiritual orientation to "living in the flow of life," she brings kindness and acceptance to whatever is happening for her.

This inspiring story shows the fruit of spiritual cultivation; it outlines the reflection inherent in it, and the quality of relationships it allows. This book is a wise companion for anyone facing a similar experience.

—WILLA THANIYA REID
(formerly Ajahn Thaniya)

"Cheryl, you should be more worried." Cheryl Wilfong's friends were puzzled by her response to a diagnosis of breast cancer. *Breast Cancer Meets Mindfulness*, a seamless blend of Dharma talk and journal, leads you through Wilfong's unexpected relationship with a condition that others perceived as a threat. She surprises us with good humor in the midst of doctors' appointments, tests, endless waiting, and surgery. The universe, she says sent her a telegram, using "one of the knockers on the front door of my body." She returns again and again to the higher truth beyond the temporal circumstance. If you're facing a personal challenge—medical or otherwise, or you're supporting a loved one who is, *Breast Cancer Meets Mindfulness* will teach you how to walk through it calmly, one mindful step at a time.

—DAWN DOWNEY, author
Stumbling Toward the Buddha: Stories about Tripping over My Principles on the Road to Transformation

Cheryl's brilliant writing helps us see and acknowledge that our suffering is part of our "common humanity" which increases our connectedness and well-being, regardless of external conditions—a huge benefit during cancer treatment, and well beyond into all areas of our life and world.

—BONNIE DURAN, Ph.D.

Cheryl has a wonderful and down-to-earth way with words. Mixed with a deep meditation practice, her writing is engaging and tells an uplifting story of surrendering to life rather than fighting with it.

— JUDSON BREWER, M.D. Ph.D. and author
The Craving Mind: From Cigarettes to Smartphones to Love — Why We Get Hooked and How We Can Break Bad Habits.

"Can cancer be funny? Is death really a humorous topic? Cheryl Wilfong's *Breast Cancer Meets Mindfulness* answers those questions with a resounding "Yes!" The charm of this book is Cheryl's realer than real approach to a perilous journey so many have had to make. With a combination of Buddhist wisdom and a refusal to succumb to self-pity, she uncovers the absurdity, the irony, and the ultimate freedom of living with a disease that if it doesn't kill you, can scare you half to death. In these compelling pages, she gives us all courage to face the unknown, and perhaps most importantly, the known."

— KEVIN GRIFFIN, author
One Breath at a Time: Buddhism and the Twelve Steps

Cheryl's dedication to meditation practice helps maintain her sense of humor, even as she manages the many challenges of her cancer diagnosis.

— JILL SHEPHERD
Insight Meditation teacher

What a surprise that something as unnerving and disruptive as a cancer diagnosis ends up being the setting for priceless discovery, the door to so much wisdom and even profound peace. This surprise awaits the reader of this delicious book. It also is there for anyone experiencing a difficult life situation, cancer or otherwise. How vividly Cheryl Wilfong portrays her own experience and insights. Compellingly (and gently) she invites the reader in to notice our own responses to scary situations—and shows how to become unshackled by them. What a blessing is *Breast Cancer Meets Mindfulness*. For it is truly about the life of being a cancer patient, and just as truly about being alive, in whatever situation we find ourselves. In an ocean of present-day books meaning to be helpful (whether about cancer or about spirituality), this one truly is. Cheryl's experience as a cancer patient revealed many things to her. We all benefit from her willingness to share them.

—JAN FRAZIER, author
   *When Fear Falls Away: The Story
   of a Sudden Awakening*

Cheryl illuminates what's essential in the Dharma, the practice of turning obstacles into doorways that lead us home.

—VINNY FERRARO
   Insight Meditation teacher

Breast Cancer Meets
Mindfulness

Surrendering to Life

ALSO BY CHERYL WILFONG

Breast Cancer Meets
Mindfulness

Surrendering to Life

CHERYL WILFONG

Cheryl Wilfong
Heart Path Press, L3C
314 Partridge Road
Putney VT 05346

www.cherylwilfong.com

Breast Cancer Meets Mindfulness

BOOK DESIGN BY CAROLYN KASPER

ISBN: 978-0-9972729-6-3

Follow Breast Cancer Meets Mindfulness *on Facebook*

This book is dedicated to Matthew Flickstein, the teacher who shows me the way to insight and non-duality.

Contents

Preface xix

ON RETREAT:
HEALING FROM SURGERY

PRO-ACTIVITY:
RADIATION

THE NEW ME: ONCOLOGY

Preface

MY LIFE TOOK an unexpected turn when I was twenty-five and I fell into a black pit. Back then I didn't know the word "depression." I knew nothing about therapy or meds. A mentor suggested that I start meditating. Seven months of daily meditation later, I was back on level ground—just barely. One thing I knew for sure: meditation had saved my suicidal life. For my thirtieth birthday, I gave myself my first ten-day meditation retreat.

When I was in my mid-fifties, my women's group had a memorable discussion in which the eight of us each talked in depth about our various spiritual paths. I said that although I went on an annual ten-day silent retreat, I yearned to go on a six-week meditation retreat. Deb, a sixty-year-old Congregational minister-in-training, said, "Tell Bill you are going, and give him a choice of when." I told my sweetie a year and a half beforehand, and I gave him a choice of when. Later, he didn't remember this conversation, but I did. I went to my first really long retreat.

Once I had my partner's initial agreement, and he became confident that he could survive without me and that I was not abandoning him, I continued to go on a month-long retreat every year, plus a handful of week-long retreats. I began to get glimpses—called *insights*—into what the Buddha says are the three characteristics of all experience:

- All things are impermanent. Everything changes. Nothing is stable.
- Unsatisfactoriness is inherent in everything—even the best things in life—when you look quite closely.
- That being said, there's nothing to hold on to. My "self" turns out to be a fiction, an unexamined assumption.

I began studying the Buddha's teachings in earnest when I was fifty. When I was sixty, Spirit Rock Meditation Center certified me to teach meditation in my local community.

By my mid-sixties, when breast cancer entered my life, I was well steeped in Buddhist studies, and that turned out to be my lifesaver—my "mindsaver"—when I was once again confronted by an unexpected turn of life. Thanks to my Buddhist meditation practice, I was able to traverse the rocky cliffs of life with a calm mind. Imagine that!

Here's the story of that journey.

PROLOGUE:
BEFORE I KNEW:
The Mammogram

Life as My Higher Power

WHEN I SCHEDULED my mammogram, I had just finished teaching a class on Mindfulness as a Higher Power. We never did get around to discussing mindfulness, but I did see that my Higher Power is karma. Karma directs my here-and-now actions, because I can see that I reap what I sow. Therefore, I need to be careful about what seeds I'm sowing in the present moment. Planting worry today forms the habit of worry tomorrow. Planting generosity now reaps the habit of openhandedness next week. Planting calm here and now teaches the mind how to rest.

Other people in the class talked about the group itself as a Higher Power. Oh yes. It's all in the company you keep, no matter who you are or how young or old you are. Behaviors, gestures, and words are all contagious. Hang out with worrywarts and you'll worry, too. Spend time with people who exercise, and you'll find yourself exercising. Go to meetings with nondrinkers, and you'll find yourself not drinking. Listen to talk shows that hate Hillary, and you'll hate Hillary, too.

Another person took Faith as her Higher Power—which is important if you're ever going to take the first step on any spiritual path. Someone took Wisdom as a Higher Power. Yes to that. I'll take more wisdom any day of the week. Someone else took Presence as their Higher Power, the nowness of now, which is all there is, really.

Even though the class is over, I'm now experimenting with Life as a Higher Power. Could I surrender to Life? Just go where Life is taking me anyway, whether or not I want it, whether or not I want to go there. Could I stop acting as if I know better than Life how to live it? Could I stop trying to control Life?

I have spent years of my life kicking and screaming against the way things are. I want circumstances to be different! Oh, how I want something different from what I'm getting. *That's not fair. That's not right. It's not supposed to be like this. I want what other people have. I want to be normal.*

But you know what? Life has actually been pretty good to me, even when I was pulling my oars in a different direction, with all my might, away from where my life stream was taking me. I could never have foreseen the good things that lay downstream in front of me, around the bend in the river. I thought I was in charge of the map. Ha! So shortsighted.

A few years ago, a meditation teacher said he didn't have a to-do list. I puzzled over that for a couple of years. How is that even possible? Little by little, though, I released my grip on my to-do list, which might as well be called a to-*be* list. That's the list of the person I want to be, the person I want to become—an organized person, a together person, a neat person, a do-everything person, a can-do person.

What if, instead of seeing myself as the doer, I simply notice Life unfolding? Some things get "done," not by my doing and not on my timetable, but just when they are somehow ready.

All I have to do is surrender to Life—my Higher Power of the month.

Life's Conveyor Belts

SOMETIMES WE PUT ourselves on conveyor belts willingly, and sometimes we find ourselves on one of life's conveyor belts with very few choices to make. All decisions are under someone else's, some other system's, control.

Flying, for instance, is a conveyor belt we willingly put ourselves on. As soon as you park your car, you've mostly lost control of your forward momentum for the next several hours. The shuttle delivers you to the terminal on its own schedule. You walk to your airline counter and stand in line, a sort of slowly moving conveyor belt, until you get to the kiosk that spits out your boarding pass. You walk to the security check and stand in line. You proceed to the slow line that scans your bags. If you are detained for a few minutes for a pat-down or someone pawing through your bags, you cannot hurry them up. You wait patiently (or not) until you get the all-clear.

While you are in the clutches of the airport, you really have no say in your movement. The conveyor belts of moving walkways can quicken your walk to your gate, where you wait. About 20 percent of the time, your plane is delayed—maybe for half an hour, maybe for four hours—and there's nothing you can do except wait patiently (or not). Sometimes you hear people ranting at the gate agent or at the person sitting next to them about the delay. They are under the mistaken assumption that complaining is effective. The conveyor belt is stopped or perhaps broken. In fact, going forward is beyond your control. Eventually you board according to some numbering system or other, you take your seat, and you sit patiently (or not) or try to sleep your way through the unpleasantness for an hour or four or twelve.

The plane lands, and you receive permission to disembark, which you do in a polite and orderly manner. If you've checked your luggage, you go to the baggage claim where you retrieve your bag from a conveyor belt. Then you follow the sign for "Ground Transportation" as you look for a bus, a car-rental desk, or a hotel shuttle. With that rent-a-car key finally in your hand, you exit the airport's giant conveyor belt, which is designed to move hundreds and thousands of people as efficiently as possible, and if one of them is you, that is your good fortune.

The hospital is another sort of conveyor belt. When you walk in through those automatic sliding glass doors, you give up your autonomy. You wait to register and then you wait in some other waiting room for the next medical receptionist to give you permission to proceed. You are waiting for someone else's schedule to intermesh with yours. Whether you're there for a routine blood test or you come in through the emergency door, a system has been designed to cover all the bases, sign all the paper work, do all the tests—not for your convenience, but for someone else's. You wait. You look at your iPhone. You wait. You page through a back issue of *People* magazine— it doesn't matter how old it is, it's still the same old news, just with different names. You wait for the doctor to see you. You go from being a person with thoughts, ideas, relationships, lists of things to do, and some authority over your life to a body with a diagnosis, with a problem that will be solved by someone else.

You wait to make your next appointment. And when you walk out the hospital's automatic doors, you are finally free.

One of the reasons you want to have an advance directive is that you don't want to be thrown onto the hospital's conveyor belt against your will. Some of us may want the hospital to pull out all the stops, but some of us want the hospital to *stop* doing what they do best—saving lives. An article entitled "How Doctors Die" reveals that when doctors know they are going to die, they do not choose to have every available treatment. They know where their disease is going, and they face in that direction.

The medical establishment excels at fixing people up, and the conveyor belt can start moving with something as simple as oxygen or a pacemaker that will not quit, and no instructions have been left to have it turned off. Add a feeding tube, which then requires a catheter, and pretty soon you need Superman to stop the speeding magic bullets of the hospital trying, against the odds, to keep a dying person alive.

The person you choose to hold your durable power of attorney for health care can make decisions when you have lost the ability to make them yourself. Your durable power of attorney is your escape hatch from the hospital conveyor belt, but you have to pack your parachute before you actually need it. If you can't speak for yourself, do you want to be attached to a lifeline? Or would you rather be able to step off the conveyor lifebelt into the terminal phase of life, called dying? Do you want someone to pull the ripcord so that you can float off into the heavens? The job of handling your durable power of attorney will be so much easier if you've left clear instructions, which means you need to be clear yourself. Now. The stakes are high. It's a matter of life (do you really want that belabored-breathing kind of "life"?) and death.

I myself am not quite ready to have DNR (Do Not Resuscitate) tattooed on my chest, but I might have AND (Allow Natural Death) tattooed on my body to speak for me when I cannot, to remind my loved ones and the hospital of what I truly desire.

Funerals are yet another form of conveyor belt. From the time the guys in suits drive a hearse into your driveway to pick up the body of your loved one who just died an hour ago, you lose control. The body bag, the gurney. Zip. Zip. The funeral home thinks it is being helpful and protecting you from the facts of death and saving you from unpleasant feelings.

They will give your loved one the same treatment that they give everyone else. The funeral home is the expert; they know how to do it; and you don't need to worry your pretty little head about a single thing. They will rewrite the lovingly handcrafted obituary you wrote into a standard format that meets newspaper guidelines and can leave out the human details of your dear one's life story.

If you ask, if you insist, you can do things "outside the box." You can dress the body, as people did a century ago. You can be present for the closing of the casket. But if you don't know, and don't ask, the funeral home will take care of it all for you, so you don't have to feel "bad." You will find yourself listening to organ Muzak with songs you don't recognize or wish you didn't recognize, and then it's over, and you feel stunned by the loss and the emptiness.

Life's institutional conveyor belts are meant to move us through certain situations on automatic pilot, so we don't have to think, so we don't have to pay attention.

Some of us willingly give over control to the professionals who must know what they are doing. Sometimes Life throws us onto a conveyor belt we hadn't planned on. But one day, our life on automatic pilot is over. And where did it go?

I wasn't even noticing.

Mammogram Follow-Up

I DO LIKE TO keep up with my various medical exams, but since insurance doesn't cover an appointment at 364 days since the one before, all my "annual" exams slide slowly, but inexorably, toward thirteen months. One year, the date for my annual mammogram had slid into Christmas Eve. However, I left the day after Christmas for a three-week vacation, so I couldn't get my mammogram until I returned. I felt slightly uneasy about the delay, but really, mid-January was the soonest I could make a date for that cold machine to squeeze my breasts.

So I went for my annual mammogram, a month "late," in mid-January. A new, young technician named Milly was making sure she did everything right. She laid my right breast on the plate and had me hug the pink machine, practically kiss the compressor as she tightened it and tightened it some more.

Radiology called me a few days later, and I went in for a second mammogram on the right breast with just a cookie-cutter-sized lens. They wanted a second look at a tiny cloud on the chest wall. A cloud that wasn't on last year's mammogram. A cloud that showed up clearly this year, thanks to Milly's dutiful squee-e-e-eezing of the plates.

Still wearing the pink hospital half-gown, I went to lie down on the ultrasound bed. How did they see what they were seeing, anyway? To me, the picture on the black-and-white monitor looked like a partly cloudy night sky. The technician ran cool gel over my right breast, zeroing in at ten o'clock. She clicked her keyboard a few times, taking pictures of various clouds, and then she escorted me into the radiologist's office next door.

Dr. Watson sat there in the dark, lit by a dozen computer monitors, comparing last year's mammogram to this year's and to today's ultrasound. He showed me what he was looking at. The striation of the muscle of the chest wall was interrupted by a barnacle, about a centimeter long and half as wide.

He walked me down one flight of stairs to the surgeons' office and asked me, "Do you have a preference for which surgeon?"

"No," I said.

"She wants an appointment with Dr. Rosen," the radiologist told the receptionist. Then he shook my hand and left. The receptionist made my appointment for the following Tuesday.

As I lay in a hospital gown on the bed in Dr. Rosen's office the following Tuesday in early February, Dr. Rosen's ultrasound monitor didn't look as high-resolution as the one in the mammography department. The screen looked all cloudy to me, but eventually he found what he was looking for, which I could barely recognize from the previous week's black-and-white photo. "I'm underwhelmed," he said. "Shall we do this?"

"Hey, I'm here," I said. "You're here. Let's proceed."

After applying a topical anesthetic, he stuck a metal shish kebab skewer into my right breast. No pain, just pressure. "You'll have a bruise," he said.

Inside the skewer was a tiny dart gun, which he fired into that centimeter-long barnacle, so it would grab a hangnail's worth of flesh. He extracted this core sample; then, warming to his game, he fired two more times. And as long as I was lying here all shimmed up with cushions and looking pretty relaxed, he fired a couple more. He then inserted a teensy-weensy titanium spiral to mark the spot.

"Titanium?" I asked.

"Airport security doesn't pick up titanium," Dr. Rosen said.

As I was checking out of the office, making my next appointment, I saw the plastic bottle with my five tiny samples leave the room with a runner, who, I assumed, was taking them to the pathology lab.

I didn't really think too much about my next appointment. Cancer doesn't run in my family. I've had other ultrasounds and biopsies of my thyroid, which turned out to be benign cysts and nodules.

On the morning of Monday, February 16, when I sat down in front of Dr. Rosen's desk, he handed me a thick paperback book with a cover design of tulips and the title *Breast Cancer*.

"You didn't bring anyone with you?" he asked.

I shook my head. He began to talk in multisyllabic words. I concentrated. I didn't allow my mind to wander.

This was the moment, the very moment, the exact moment when years of mindfulness practice paid off.

In meditation, we choose a meditation object for the foreground of our attention. Often enough, the breath or body sensation or hearing slides to the background as the puppy mind runs away. Moment after moment, we bring our meditation object back to the foreground. That's what I did now, sitting in front of the surgeon—keeping my mind focused on the meditation object of hearing and comprehending what he was saying.

After an hour and a half, I understood the game plan, though I couldn't repeat the details of the whys and wherefores to Bill or any of my friends.

Surgery—a lumpectomy—in ten days. He would take out at least three lymph nodes. Immediate pathology reports would tell him whether he would need to take more. And then I would wait for a month to heal.

I stopped at the receptionist's desk, and she made a list of the things I needed to do: blood test, urinalysis, chest x-ray, and EKG. She made an appointment for a breast MRI on Friday.

I walked downstairs and within an hour had done the blood test, the urinalysis, the chest x-ray, and the EKG.

Then I walked out of the hospital into a clear, blue, cold, and beautiful February day.

AND THEN . . .
Diagnosis & Surgery

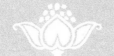

Entrances to Holiness

Entrances to holiness are everywhere.
— Shabbat Morning Prayer Book

MY ENTRANCE TO holiness opened on Monday, February 16, when the surgeon handed me a thick booklet entitled *Breast Cancer*. I entered the holy place of fearlessness. For the succeeding hour and a half, as I sat in front of Dr. Rosen at his desk, I strained to understand everything he was saying. I made my decisions—the ones that could be made that day—and walked out with a surgery date ten days hence, *if* there were no glitches.

I hadn't brought anyone with me because I really thought the biopsy report would be negative. I was healthy. I was active. I ate well. I had a good immune system.

Those thought balloons popped in rapid succession to reveal the signboard behind them: I am mortal. *Pop!* went the thought of *Not me, not now. Sssss* went the balloon of *I have a good immune system.*

I couldn't repeat to my friends what the surgeon had said with so many multisyllabic words, but I had confidence in him and in Brattleboro Memorial Hospital. After I left his office, I had a blood test, urinalysis, a chest x-ray, and an EKG within the following hour. That was fast. That was efficient. That was easy. That was stress-free. The conveyor belt of the hospital system worked really well that afternoon.

I had entered the house of wholeness, of surrendering to Life's plan for me. What could I control anyway? Not much. I could ask questions, advocate for myself, and call my best friend-nurse, Barbara.

My mind stayed in the present—a not-tense place. My friends began to worry, to recommend their remedies to me. My friends were afraid.

I remained in the presence of the present, not seeking to know the unknowable future. Content with the holy place of Now. Not wishing for anything different than what Life was delivering.

Meet the Heavenly Messengers

SUSPECTED I HAD been skating on thin ice. After all, I was in my mid-sixties. Well, okay, late sixties. Bodies deteriorate. Something was bound to happen. In the meantime, I was resting on my laurels. Not that they were "my" laurels, but my thoughts acted as if I were the one responsible for my good health. After all, I ate well, I exercised, I lived a clean life. Then I went to the surgeon.

Really, the cracks in the ice were becoming rather loud—two mammograms, an ultrasound, a biopsy—but I continued in the denial of *Not me, surely*, skating right out to the edge of that thin ice. Breast cancer.

Aging, disease, and death—the teachings of the Buddha call these facts of life the "Heavenly Messengers." How can the hard facts of life be "heavenly"? Because these three unpleasant realities have the potential to jolt me awake to my life. This possibility of waking up is the fourth heavenly messenger.

In the legend of the Buddha's life, the twenty-nine-year-old Buddha-to-be was shocked and disgusted by seeing, for the first time, an old person, then a sick person, and finally a dead person lying on the side of the road. Being of the warrior class, he felt it was unfitting for him to flinch in the face of aging, sickness, and death. Then he saw an ascetic walking serenely among these unpleasantries.

We, too, are face to face with aging, illness, and ceasing, even deceasing, every day. If we have the nerve to look, really look, these ordinary, everyday envoys alert us to the existential realities we would prefer to avoid.

Actually, aging, disease, and death are not our enemies; they are our allies in living our own true life. The deepest regret that dying people have is that they did not pursue their dreams and aspirations but instead settled for what people expected of them. Knowing that our time is short, even if we expect to have twenty or fifty more years, now is the time to live our very own truth. Now is the time to be true to our self. These Heavenly Messengers of aging, disease, and death can give us the courage to get down to the business of living our very own "wild and precious life."

Until we come face to face with the deep questions of our own existence, most of us don't want to be contaminated with aging, illness, and death. When some of my friends hear me talking about aging or hospice—again—they roll their eyes. "Puh-lease, Cheryl. TMI. Why do you talk about this so much? Can't you talk about something pleasant?"

The Heavenly Messengers of aging, illness, and death are not ethereal beings and they don't look like angels—except, perhaps, the angel of death. These messengers are of this earth and may look quite ugly or germy or repulsive. They are the natural unfolding of life; there is nothing supernatural about them. These divine envoys carry an important and urgent message for our minds: our bodies are mortal.

I read the text of my message—cancer—and understood the subtext of the message—my body is now old. In fact, this disease may be my entry point into old age. I have passed all the other milestones: retirement, senior discounts, Social Security, and Medicare. Now comes the nail in the coffin (ahem), my body has a disease—cancer. The cancer in my breast is very small, but cancer can kill people. Now, with the disease of cancer, I myself have become a heavenly messenger.

In my daily life, I really prefer to accent youth, health, and life. Who wouldn't? Youth is so much more beautiful than age; health is a lot more comfortable than sickness; and, of course, I prefer life to the alternative.

Thanks to my trapeze and acrobatic classes at the circus school, my body is firmer and more toned than it has ever been. Aside from cancer, I am healthy. These mental gymnastics are what they call *denial*. After all, I am always the oldest person in my circus classes.

Breast cancer. The Heavenly Messengers delivered a telegram, and they used one of the knockers on the front door of my body.

My brother was a UPS driver in Florida for a couple of years. He got calluses on his right hand's knuckles from knocking on the doors of retirees. My challenge is to not be callous toward the aging and aged in my life. Now, that includes me. No more believing that "sixty is the new forty" or telling myself, "Gee, Cheryl, you don't look your age," or "Don't worry, Cheryl, you're going to live for a long time yet."

The thin ice of the aging body has cracked and revealed the flow of life underneath. Once, Bill and I were ice skating on the West River in the rare condition of black ice. The ice had frozen crystal clear, like glass. It looked as if I was skating on water; I could see the bottom of the river under my feet. I kept feeling very anxious about falling into the frozen water, even though the ice was several inches thick. A muskrat darted through the water below me. Now I see disease, life, and death very clearly.

This river of aging has eddies and backwaters, but also fast currents of illness. I may float down that river quickly or slowly. Maybe I will dally along the near shore for some while yet. Still, this river of life flows on, emptying out, I know, into the great ocean. And I can almost see that ocean on the horizon, getting closer every day.

Wake up, Cheryl. Wake up to life.

Barbara, RN

WHEN I RETURNED home after hearing my diagnosis, the first person I e-mailed was Barbara, RN (Retired Nurse). I'm slowly beginning to realize that a nurse can never really retire. Barbara's always on call for her friends. She's been a blessing to our women's group. When Fritze learned she had colorectal cancer, Barbara went with her for the surgical implantation of Fritze's chemo port. When Deb's lung function suddenly fell exceedingly low, Barbara went with her to one doctor's appointment, and spoke with Deb often because of the mysterious nature of Deb's illness. Now I e-mailed Barbara to ask if she could come to my next doctor's appointment with me.

In 2002, while four of us were taking a day hike near Chesterfield, New Hampshire, we came back to the parking lot to find Barbara's passenger-side window smashed. Two of our four pocketbooks had been stolen. None of us had cell phones in those days. While three of us were still trying to comprehend what had happened, Barbara disappeared. She went to find the nearest house, which, when I looked down the road in both directions, was invisible to me. Chesterfield's only town police car arrived about five minutes later, and Barbara returned. That's how I know that Barbara is good in an emergency.

My dear Bill, on the other hand, seems like a deer in the headlights. His mental clutch is in, and his mental gears do not engage for a while. He's a good companion, but he's a distracted navigator when the pressure is on. I rely on Bill for hugs, but I rely on Barbara for her sharp and scientific mind.

With Bill, I am often the strong one, the organized one. But Barbara is an alpha; she takes the lead when we are hiking. With Barbara in charge, I can relax—I can even fall apart if I need to, thanks to Barbara's healing touch.

I Have Cancer
All Over My Body

THE DAY AFTER I heard my diagnosis, breast cancer, I woke up with the thought, *I've got cancer all over my body and I don't know it.*

For the past fifteen years, I've had cysts and nodules on my thyroid. I go to the endocrinologist every two or three years for a checkup, and she tells me my cysts and nodules grow a millimeter or two a year. She says that, in case they turn malignant, thyroid cancer is a slow-growing cancer. But wait! When was the last time I saw Dr. Shields? Four years ago! A lot can happen in four years. Her office was supposed to call me for a follow-up last year! But they didn't.

I called for an appointment. "Since we haven't seen you in more than three years, you'll have to get a referral from your doctor." *Wait a minute. That's not fair. It's your fault that your office hasn't seen me.*

I called my doctor. The soonest she could see me was the day after my lumpectomy. I made that appointment. Then I was still stuck with my mind and that stressful thought: *I've got cancer all over my body, and I don't know it.*

A thought like this is disturbing. A thought like this causes suffering. I know from experience not to believe all my thoughts, but stopping a belief in its tracks is hard. The first step on the Buddha's Noble Eightfold Path is Wise View. Any view, any belief, any attitude that causes suffering is unwise, but how can I possibly turn this train of thought around? This train of thought, which is relentlessly chugging its way through my mind. One skillful means I can use not only to reduce stress but to actually eliminate suffering is to question a stressful thought, using an inquiry process developed by Byron Katie.

Katie, as she is called, had been depressed for ten years when she suddenly "woke up," and all suffering disappeared from her life. People began arriving on her doorstep for help. Instead of listening to their stories about each particular anguish, she asked them instead to write down each stressful thought. She developed a process of four questions and three "turn-arounds," which are opposite thoughts to the original thought.

I sat down on the sofa with my iPad and opened Byron Katie's "The Work" app. I typed in the short form of that stressful thought: *I've got cancer all over my body.* Then the app asked me the four questions.

Question 1: Is that true?

Hmmm. Well, I don't know for sure if it's true.

Question 2: Is that really true?

Since I have to answer "yes" or "no," I typed in *No.*

I cannot absolutely know for sure that it's true, even though this thought was sticking like Velcro. "Hey, pay attention to me!" This thought was acting as if it were the only thought in the world.

Question 3: How do I react when I believe that thought?

I feel scared and anxious, because I want to know the answer, but I don't know the answer.

Question 4: Who would I be without this thought?

If I didn't believe this thought, I would feel relaxed. I would focus on the good things that are happening. I would feel grateful for Bill and for all the good medical care I am receiving. If I couldn't believe this thought, I would be living in the present moment instead of trying to ratchet up the future. If I couldn't believe this thought, I would see the diagnosis of cancer as an opportunity to deepen my Dharma practice.

Then it was time for the turnarounds. These are opposite thoughts, which are also true, and actually sometimes truer than the original browbeating thought.

I don't have cancer all over my body.

Well, yes, I can be pretty sure I don't have cancer in my little finger or big toe. It's probably not in my legs or my arms. As far as I know, it is true that I do not have cancer all over my body.

I have anti-cancer all over my body.

Well, I've always thought I had a good immune system. I live a clean life and eat a pretty good diet.

Cancer has me all over my body.

Well, yes. That's true. The *idea* of cancer is whipping my mind around, running my mind all over my body (my torso really), wondering if I have cancer here or there. I could even say that cancer, the thought of cancer, has me by the throat, where my thyroid is.

I went back to the original thought: *I have cancer all over my body.*

Hey! We all have micro-cancers all over our bodies. Everyone has cancer all over their body. Mostly, our immune systems take care of these tiny cancers.

Seeing that these other three opposite (or turned-around) thoughts were equally as true as the original stressful thought that was bullying me, my mind let go. My mind relaxed.

Ahhh. Peace and quiet.

True and Not True

I'VE NOTICED SOMETHING interesting about the hamster wheel of the mind when it gets going on a repeated thought like *I'm going to die from cancer.* Around and around it goes, and I feel worse and worse. Angry frustrated, sad, afraid, whatever.

On one of my long retreats, I kept an eye on one of those repeated thoughts. Here's what I saw: a thought arises, then the thought crumbles, and there's a small gap—very easy to miss if you're not looking. The same thought repeats, and this is where I am fooled. It's the same thought, but it's not the same thought. It's the same thought, but it's a different same thought. It's a photocopied thought. It's actually another thought, like the refrain of "ninety-nine bottles of beer on the wall." It sounds like the same thought; it feels like the same thought; but it's taking place at a different time, maybe just one second later than the previous thought, which is actually dead and gone.

After watching this thought-space-thought-space-thought-space routine for a while, I began to wonder why the thought needed to repeat itself. I'd gotten the message the first time around, but the mind had launched into its own rendition of "Ninety-Nine Bottles." It was drunk on fury or worry or sadness, but the loud repetitious song kept me distracted from actually feeling those feelings.

Sometimes I ask meditation students, "What does truth feel like?" "Huh?" they respond. I don't intend this question as a koan, I really mean what does truth feel like in your body? How do you know something is true? What does "true" feel like?

Sometimes, a student thinks of a fact, like divorce, and calls truth "hard." I am not angling for the hard facts, though I love facts of all sorts.

Sit back. Relax. How do you know when something is true?

Truth makes my mind relax. Truth quiets my mind, maybe for an entire second. Maybe for two or three seconds. *Ahhh. Oh. Mmmm.* My body relaxes. Calm arrives. Sometimes truth makes the hairs on my arms stand up; sometimes truth gives me goosebumps.

Like the time Hope told me about going to Alaska to visit her son when she was sixty. One afternoon, she said, she took a sightseeing flight, and the engine conked out. As the plane was coasting down to the forested mountains, Hope looked out the window and thought to herself, "Well, I've had a good life."

When I heard that, I got goosebumps. That's what truth feels like. Knowing in your bones that something is true to the depth of your being. No questions asked.

Miraculously, rescue arrived an hour after Hope's

plane went down. None of the five passengers was seriously injured.

So then, what's going on with the hamster-wheel mind? Thought-space-repeated thought-space. Here I am believing that stressful thought, but if that thought were true, my mind would be quiet. Actually, it's that tiny space between thoughts that's the truth. The mind needs to repeat itself because it's telling itself a lie, trying to teach the mind an untruth. *Repeat after me.* When I believe that hamster-wheel thought, I am believing a lie for a second. Then the mind can't sustain the lie and collapses into half a second of silence. If that stressful thought were truly true, the mind wouldn't have to tell me again. And again. If the mind repeats the lie often enough, will I believe it?

Truth is right here in the present moment. I need go no further. Simply notice that the mind stops. Stop. Go. Stop. Go.

Can I stop believing the go-go-go of the mind? Can I surrender to truth?

The Universe

FOR YEARS, I referred to The Universe as my arbiter of life. God was dead for me; He died when I was sixteen, and I never could resuscitate the relationship. So, in a conversation, when a Christian or Jew or Moslem might refer to God or Allah, I would say "The Universe."

I would chalk up the unknown, the unplanned, and surprises of all sorts to The Universe. My casual relationship to The Universe was not at all personal. Days and weeks would go by without me giving The Universe a single thought. The Universe may sound big, but what I actually believed in, on a daily basis, was the agency of my self. All day long, my mind was filled with things done by Me—the doer, of course. I was arranging the world, my every day, exactly as I wanted it. Each day, another day of me, me, and me. I, me, mine.

Oh, The Universe threw me plenty of curveballs. *No! I don't want that! That's not the way it should be.* My resistance to life was driven by the strong belief in the little god of Me, with only fleeting references, a quick nod of the head, to The Universe.

Then, in my mid-fifties, I began to pray: *May I see*

things as they really are. May I see and accept things as they really are happening.

By the time breast cancer entered my life when I was sixty-seven, enough wisdom had lodged under the rocks and between the stones of the river of life that I could finally say: I surrender. I surrender to Life as it is. For I no longer called it The Universe—that huge, amorphous everything. I had converted. Now I called it Life. Life was alive, a felt presence.

By this time, I had actually seen and felt Life once. I call it my unborn day. The day I was unborn of my self for half an hour. The day the river of Life flowed through my eyes, and I saw that it never has been me doing the seeing. Seeing is only Life looking at itself. The day I saw that death of the body was only another expression of life, and really not that important. So amazing. So impossible to put into words.

I've been floating in the river of life all along, but now I am keenly aware of it. It's a mesmerizing ride. There's no need for me to argue or complain. No need to have an opinion. No need to judge.

Life unfolding. Here. Now.

The Future Is Just an Idea

I TEACH MEDITATION AT least once a week, and sometimes three times a week. Hundreds of times I've heard myself say:

> *Label that thought "past" or "future."*
> *Notice that a thought of the past is a thought. It is just a thought. The past is only an idea.*
> *The body is always in the present moment, the only place it ever can be.*
> *Notice that a thought of the future is a thought. It is just a thought. The future is only an idea that we have, and then we believe it. The future is a thought happening in the present moment.*
> *The body-mind remains in the present moment.*

Once in a while, I actually understand that the future is just an idea, just my imagination playing games with me.

Here I was, with a diagnosis of cancer, living my ordinary, daily life. I could keep my mind on what I was doing right now—say, snowshoeing in the woods—or I could let my mind run ahead and pay more attention to the movie in my mind than the squirrel tracks in the snow. Reality? Or virtual reality? The reality of my five senses here and now? Or the unreality of my mind? Cold breeze, body beginning to perspire on the uphill, bare trees, mouse tracks in the snow, and the joy of being outdoors? Or thoughts of cancer, doctors, hospitals, disease, and, scariest of all, death?

The choice really is mine, even though it doesn't feel like a choice, even though my mind runs off to the future like an untrained puppy.

One definition of mindfulness is tethering the mind to the body; we could say tethering the mind to the present moment, since the body is always in the present moment. For most of my life, I have let my mind wander wherever it wants, to whatever playground it wishes. I have loved my mind and its creativity. But now is the time to take the puppy mind to obedience school. *Stay. Stay in the present moment.*

The body is right here, right now. When the mind wanders off to the future, it's just an idea. The body can never experience the future. The body can never be in the future. The body-mind stays right here in the present moment. The future is an idea in the mind. The mind has an idea—of the future, for instance—and then it believes that idea. When you stop to think about it, the future is an idea happening in the present moment. How sneaky is that!

The future is as real as a rainbow, something we are always chasing after, yet can never reach. We can never live somewhere over the rainbow because we are always right here, right now.

You can see and hear the past and future in some sort of murky, vague way—in your mind. Yet hearing and seeing in your imagination are never as sharp as they are in the present moment, when all your seeing-hearing-touching-tasting-smelling senses are perfectly clear and available.

The vague images and imperfectly imagined future conversations (perhaps with ourselves) stir up our emotions, and that's how past and future grab us and cling to us. That's how we make up the story of our self—our "I am."

Past and future are the ideas out of which I spin the story of my self. These ideas of past and future constitute the story line of my life. My past defines my self. Memory of the past is what makes me "me." After all, my past is mine, and not anyone else's.

Yet the past is an idea, a product of the imagination. The future is an idea. Past and future are all in my head. Really, I may as well be here now, because it's the only place I ever can be. What if life is just a string of present moments—without a string?

Really, really, all I have is this present moment with a foam of bubbles—my past, my future—each bubble popping to be quickly replaced by another bit of foam in the mindstream. You have to finely tune your mindfulness to notice this wonderful illusion.

The future is a dream, a daydream. Stop daydreaming

and wake up to the present moment. Stop sleepwalking through life. Wake up to your here-and-now life. This day. This now. Now.

Now.

The Future Is Always
a Stressful Idea

When I introduce new students to brief meditations on hearing, on body sensations, or on breath, I ask, "What did you notice?" Someone always says, "I feel so calm." Or "I feel relaxed." It's a surprising discovery: Peace is in the present moment.

Past and future are both stressful. Past and future are both stressful *ideas*. Distress, plain and simple. I can certainly recognize the stress of anxiety and worry—not knowing what the future will bring, and fearing that it will be bad.

Planning is another very common form of thinking about the future. Of course, planning can be useful, but it is really useless to overdo the planning. I was astounded when a meditation teacher referred to a quote from the Buddha: "A wise person thinks any thought she wants to think, and doesn't think any thought she doesn't want to think."* The teacher talked about planning to pack for a

---

* Vassakara Sutta.

transatlantic flight. "I review my packing list once," she said. "And then I'm done."

Wow! I could free up a lot of bandwidth if I reduced planning—for anything—to a once-over.

Thanks to my many retreats, I have managed to shorten my view of the future to a day or two. I don't think about packing until the day before I leave home. Bill wants me to stay at home to help him pack his roller bag. "Bill," I say, "I'm packed." I take one of each—short-sleeved shirt, three-quarter-sleeved shirt, long-sleeved shirt, jacket, shorts, capri pants, long pants, swimsuit, and an all-purpose meditation shawl. Two sets of underwear, two pairs of socks, and two pairs of shoes. Done. I'm going out to the garden to play.

Bill, poor dear, spends a couple of hours stressing over packing this-or-that or this-*and*-that, as if there is a right choice and a wrong choice. Really, how many times do you want to plan your suitcase? What, pray tell, is the use of stressing out over the unknown future?

Anticipation is thinking about a positive future—I look forward to a good thing. Even so, my body responds to this good stress, this eustress, as stress. Excitement about a lover, a baby, a vacation, a new something-or-other creates tension in the body. It feels like fun. Desire can feel great. And it is stressful.

All these different forms of futuring are taking place in the mind. It's all happening in the virtual reality of imagination, and each future—negative or positive—is stressful.

Sometimes, I find my mind reviewing the things I need to do tomorrow. *Cheryl*, I say to myself, *you know how to go grocery shopping. You don't need to think about it more than once.* Things will happen as they happen. Really, I don't need to over-plan grocery shopping or going to the post office or what streets I'm going to take to get there. My body, my intuition, my knowing will make those decisions then. It's a waste of energy to make them now—again and again.

The past is gone. Gone. Reviewing the unpleasant past with regret, reliving embarrassment, shame, or trauma is stressful, of course.

In the past, I didn't have cancer. Or so I thought. Comparing that past to today's present is stressful as well as useless.

Even reviewing the *pleasant* past is stressful, because when you wake up from that daydream, it's over and done. That pleasant thing has come to an end, and is, in fact, no longer available. Sigh. That sigh is the body releasing stress.

After all these years of mindfulness mind-training, my mind often happily stays in the present moment— a place of no stress. A place of peace. No desire to be anywhere else, any time else. Here, today, this moment, the only moment there ever is.

Notice Where, Somewhere in Your Body, Something Relaxes

ANOTHER MEDITATION instruction I frequently offer is this:

> *As you return your attention to the present moment,*
> *notice where, somewhere in your body,*
> *something relaxes.*

Each and every thought causes tension in my body. It may be only a tiny tension, but for that moment of anxiety, sadness, or irritation, my body is ready to fight, flee, or freeze. My body is ready to save itself, while my mind churns up a story. *I'm going to die. It's not fair. That's not right.*

Pause. Take a break. Bring your attention to your breath. Your body is breathing. As that stressful thought fades a bit, notice where, somewhere in the body, something relaxes.

For me, it's my left shoulder and my left buttock.

It could be a tiny muscle under the eye. Or your throat. My left hand is grasping my leg so lightly that it's easy to miss. Maybe it's your thigh. Or your jaw. Notice that something relaxes.

Breathe.

Hearing Rest

TEN YEARS AGO, thirty-year-old Talia told me that, as a result of living in Japan and going to temples every weekend to meditate, she had learned how to still her mind. I looked at her in disbelief. Did she apply vise-grips of will to hold her mind in place? Did she glue her mind in place with rock-solid intention? Did she grit her teeth and strong-arm her thoughts into submission?

I should have known that the answer, as always, is simple mindfulness.

Eventually, I received guidance from Shinzen Young, who spent three years as a monk in a Vajrayana Zen monastery in Japan in his early twenties. In the mid-1970s, he returned to Los Angeles, where he grew up, and, at age twenty-six, lived at the International Buddhist Meditation Center with a couple dozen other meditation teachers of all persuasions. As he says, "I was walking around with a big stick, and the insight meditation teachers were getting all the students." Some Zen teachers whack sleepy students between the shoulder blades with a pliable stick, like a slat from a wooden venetian blind, except wider. This whack wakes them up. Needless to say, the stick looked daunting to American students of meditation.

Shinzen soon went to Australia to sit a two-month retreat with U Pandita, a Burmese monk who was called "the teacher of teachers." Thus, for the past forty years, Shinzen has been teaching mindfulness.

Shinzen has a unique noting system—that is, for taking note, paying attention to exactly what is happening in any given moment. Here's my version of part of it.

> *Notice hearing. Simply notice sounds arising and passing away.*
> *Label these sounds by whispering to yourself in your mind, "Hearing. Hearing."*
> *We are not paying attention to what the sound is, although our perception faculty will jump right in and say, "Bird singing" or "Door closing." We are paying attention simply to hearing.*
> *The mind will wander away like a little puppy. Although we usually call that "thinking," we could also call it "hearing in"—hearing the internal world.*
> *We return our attention to "hearing out"—hearing the external world.*
> *If we become aware of quietude or the sound of silence or the tiny space between thoughts, we can call that "hearing rest."*

Sometimes, Shinzen directs us to notice "talk space." Where, in your head, do you feel your mind talking to you? (Some people who are entirely visual thinkers "see" their thoughts, and have very little "talk" going on.)

You can begin by noticing the space at or between the ears. For me, "talk space" is somewhere behind the left sinus under my eye, but it will be different for everyone. I really enjoy focusing on "talk space" and noticing how thoughts, now called "hearing in," very subtly vibrate that area. In fact, when I focus on my "talk space," and use "hear rest" to label my experience, mind chatter quiets down to occasional static with wisps of words and thoughts. For the past couple of years, "hearing rest" has been my favorite meditation object. Calm and contentment are the easiest positive emotions for me to access, and the quieted mind is quite relaxing. Tranquility descends over my body. Not only does the mind come to rest, the body also rests. Freed of the tiny tensions generated by each and every thought, I begin to embody peace and relaxation.

Notice that I arrived in this still place not through force of will, but simply through mindfulness. Sometimes, of course, the mind just does not quiet down, so I have plenty of opportunities for noticing "hearing in."

Eventually, these few seconds of "hearing rest" spill over into my everyday activities. Taking a walk, I notice a few seconds of quiet mind, where I am simply walking and hearing birdsong. Driving the car (my radio is always off), I tune in to a few seconds of silent mind and feel more alert than usual. In the middle of the night, in bed with an attack of restless legs, I turn my attention to "hear rest," and, if I can keep my attention there, with intention, the restless legs calm down. If I begin to think, the restlessness flares up again. I tell you truly, "hear rest" seems like a miracle cure for those bothersome restless legs.

Having become acquainted with this space of "hear rest" and comfortable with quietude was extremely helpful when I received the diagnosis of breast cancer. I could notice the few occasions when my mind went galloping off to some dire possibility, and rein it in. I could then give myself a little pep talk on the uselessness of worry. The mind wants to know the unknowable future. It wants to know, wants to know, wants to know. I would remind myself that not even the doctor knew, not even the expert knew truly, what the next step would be. Oh, they had their educated guesses, which had a high probability of being accurate, but really, truly, at this moment they did not know. If the doctor didn't know, I could not know. I may as well relax into the nowness of now and enjoy the beautiful day, enjoy my friends, enjoy Bill. And notice the restfulness of the present moment.

"I'm Not Worried"

KEN, A WARMHEARTED, wild-haired eighty-year-old who didn't own a comb, discovered a melanoma on the bottom of his foot. Soon thereafter, it and four of his toes were removed. The next time I saw Ken, I said, "Oh, Ken. I've been so worried about you."

"I'm not worried," he replied.

That brought me up short. He was right. No need to worry. As Shantideva, an eighth-century Buddhist monk, said, "If the problem can be solved, why worry? If the problem cannot be solved, worrying will do you no good."

Ken felt he was on a great adventure. Although he was a world traveler and spoke (and taught) Spanish, hobbling around and living his life to the fullest was part of his great adventure. He died just before his eighty-first birthday.

When I talk about surrendering to Life, I imagine one of the rivers near where I grew up in the Midwest—flat and meandering. Perhaps Ken's sense of adventure is more accurate, though.

My greatest adventure so far has been rafting the Colorado River through the Grand Canyon. The Colorado is a pool-and-drop river. After a mile or five of placid water, it is then intersected by a creek from a side canyon, which has washed boulders into the river, creating rapids. For the first many miles the rapids are fun and exciting, sort of like our lives in our teens and twenties. Then, after you've passed the midpoint of Phantom Ranch, the first and last possibility for walking out of the canyon, you hit the biggest rapids—Granite, Crystal, and finally Lava—all of which are terrifying to think about, but thrilling to experience.

One person on our trip was so anxious and worried about the river that he finally had to be helicoptered out. It really is useless to worry yourself sick.

When you receive a diagnosis of cancer, you are not going to be helicoptered out of your situation. Nor can you go back upstream, to your pre-cancer life. You can go with the flow and enjoy the adventure, or you can worry about what lies beyond the next bend, believing that whatever it is, it will be bad.

Bathing in the muddy Colorado River water, Bill felt he just couldn't get clean. He felt anxious about his back going out on the bumpety-bump-*smack* at the end of every rapid. Just upstream of Crystal Rapid, he was sick with an intestinal bug, so he spent the afternoon lying in the shade of a tree near a rattlesnake. Meanwhile, I hiked up Crystal Creek with others on our tour, and I stood under a five-foot waterfall to let the warm green water pour over my hot body.

At the end of Sapphire Rapid, the guide steering the

raft needs to make a sharp right turn. Our newish guide didn't quite make it, and the front rim of the raft began to ride up the flat rock face directly in front of us as the stern of the raft was pushed by the force of the rushing river behind us.

"High side!" she yelled as she dropped her oars and launched herself through the air, to land splat on the high front rim of the raft at the same time as did Bill and I, who were sitting in the "front seats." The raft was about to flip over, but with our combined weight of 400 pounds lying on the high side of the front rim, the raft slid off the rock face, back into the water, and away we quickly floated while the guide regained her oars.

I am not surrendering my life raft in Sapphire Rapid. I am throwing all my weight into mindfulness of the present moment. Worry about the future and what comes next is useless. My raft may flip, or maybe it won't. I may be thrown out of my raft into deep water. Or maybe I won't.

The guides instructed us that if we were thrown out of our boat and into the white water of the rapids, we should float feet-first downriver. I wasn't thrown out; I was hanging onto the raft for dear life with my feet wedged tightly between the bottom of the rim and the floor of the boat as we left the last tongue of smooth water and entered the washing machine of the next rapids.

The Buddha calls the Dharma a raft with which to cross the river of suffering. The rocky river of stress and distress can shake a person up pretty badly. I have been a student of the Dharma for twenty years, and now is the moment to put my practice into practice. All these years of noticing the small stresses, the paper cuts of daily life, with a few doozies thrown in for good measure, have enabled me to build up my muscles of "kindfulness"— mindfulness plus kindness toward the present moment, and, more importantly, kindness toward myself. All these years of noticing stress and distress, heartache and heartbreak, pains in the neck and hard knocks, have attuned my recognition of the many, many flavors of suffering, from mild to heavy. As a result, I know this one thing: when I resist, I suffer; when I let go of resistance and go with the flow of the moment, I find calm—sometimes even happiness.

Mostly, I am floating at ease in the river of life. But there are times when I am pulled through a rocky section of life, when I hang onto my Dharma raft for dear life, when I practice mindfulness, when I pause, when I practice self-compassion, or when I repeat home-made mottos or A.A.-type slogans to remind myself of my own insights or those insights I have borrowed from my meditation teachers.

We're all on a grand adventure, and it's a once-in-a-lifetime opportunity.

Friendly? Or Hostile?

MUCH OF MY attitude toward life depends on my answer to this question: *Is the universe friendly, or is it hostile?*

You can answer the question theoretically for yourself. If you decide to answer it pragmatically, then your choices are (1) the universe is hostile (notice that if you believe this, you suffer); or (2) the universe is friendly (notice that when you believe *this*, you don't suffer). The choice is yours.

Worry depends on (1) believing there is a future, and (2) believing that something bad is going to happen in that future. Worriers believe that something bad is going to happen in the future—but if the universe is essentially a friendly place, how could that ever be?

The Buddha was a homeless wanderer. He called everyone he met "friend." Could I call everyone and every situation I meet "friend"? Could I call cancer "friend"?

Bill makes friends wherever he goes. Sometimes that's his definition of a good day—*I met a new friend today.* I soon realized that Bill and I have different definitions of *friend.* I'm talking about a lifelong commitment to a particular person; he's talking about someone he met today whom he may never see again in his life. In this way, Bill is like a three-year-old at the playground who doesn't need to know his new friend's name, what he does, or anything about him. Bill is just having fun with this person, playing with them, or enjoying their company for a few minutes.

If I made a friend out of every person and every situation I meet, then I'd be living in a friendly world. Believe you me, this is not the way I was brought up.

If I believe the universe is friendly, I'd never have to be mad at life, the universe, and everything. I don't necessarily have to believe there's a reason for something happening (there isn't)—I can just be patient and curious about what's happening. I don't have to assign a personality to The Universe. *Oh, The Universe must have wanted it this way.* I simply stand on the ever-changing edge of now and watch it unfold.

The doctor tells me I have cancer. *How is this friendly?* you ask. *How is this unfriendly?* I ask.

I wouldn't choose this diagnosis of cancer, yet what can I do about it? I do what needs to be done, and then I let it be. I'll say one thing: I'm meeting new friends at the hospital every time I go there.

Surrendering Military Metaphors

W HAT'S WITH ALL the military metaphors? The *war* on cancer. I'm going to *fight* this cancer. Her *struggle* with cancer. Cancer *invades* my body. Cancer is the *enemy*. I'm going to *beat* this cancer. As any six-year-old can tell you, wars and battles mean someone is going to die.

Do I *have* to "fight" cancer? Taking a military stance toward cancer is shooting the messenger, shooting the heavenly messenger. *By God, I am not going to get old. I'm going to whip this cancer. They say I'm going to die, but I refuse to believe it.* The heavenly messenger is knocking on my door. The Heavenly Messengers deliver their telegrams of aging, illness, death, and ongoing continuous change. I, for one, want to read those messages, but I have heard many stories of people who just didn't want to hear the so-called bad news.

Is cancer really the enemy? Or is my body the enemy? Has my body betrayed me? Or is it my mind that's the culprit, putting up the resistance? Actually, the body has no opinion about cancer. The body is. Cancer is. The mind has plenty of opinions, including fighting cancer, which sounds like a sure-fire recipe for stress.

Casting the experience of cancer into "win" or "lose" leaves no room for the middle ground where many people with cancer live. Mike's father lived with prostate cancer for twenty years. Evelyn has lived with lymphoma for twenty years. My neighbor, Rich, lived with metastasized colon cancer for more than two years.

You can say Rich lost the battle in the end, but we are all going to lose the battle, one way or another. When you look at it that way, *lose* loses its meaning. Simply put, Rich died of cancer. We all have to die of something.

I could say that Rich won every day of his two-plus years of living with cancer. He played soccer every week and went to his law office every day for two years while having standard chemotherapy and then various experimental chemotherapies. Rich had the constitution of a horse. Toward the end, he had three months of failing health. That sounds like living to me, neither winning nor losing.

When a stressful thought arrives, for a few seconds, the body prepares to defend itself from stress. The body doesn't know the difference between a saber-toothed tiger that threatened our ancestors and a paper tiger that worries our modern minds. The body prepares to defend itself—fight, flight, or freeze. These are the responses of the amygdala, our reptilian brain. That ancient brain will do everything it can to protect us, to make sure we survive to another day. Its basic instinct is fear, plain and simple.

Based on fear, some of us fight cancer; others deny or doubt it (flee from the scary idea); some of us just feel helpless (freeze).

The practice of mindfulness calms the old lizard brain so that you have greater access to your mammalian brain and to your primate mind. I mean, really, do you want to act like a lizard? Or like a human being?

For me, these metaphors of fight-and-struggle against cancer go against the grain of life, yet I am choosing the word *surrender*. Surrender sounds like I am waving a white flag of defeat. I give up. But what I am giving up is the fight. I am giving up resistance to life as it is unfolding.

Since my first reading of the *Tao Te Ching*, forty years ago, I have been intrigued by one verse in particular: *Yield and overcome.** By yielding a "battle" with cancer, I overcome my fear. I sit in an open field, a former battlefield, perhaps, where a lone heavenly messenger walks serenely. As Rumi says, "Out beyond ideas of wrongdoing and rightdoing, there is a field. I'll meet you there."

I'll meet you there, too—in the openness and acceptance of Life, just as it is.

---

* *Tao Te Ching*, verse 22.

Surrendering to Life #1

I SAY I AM surrendering to Life. Life with a capital L. Not my little, mundane, supposedly individual life, but the big Life that some people call God. For me, Life is God without the personality of godliness. Life is both-ness, and-ness, all-ness. Zorba the Greek called it the "full catastrophe." It is what it is, and it is *as* it is.

In A. A., this attitude is epitomized by the Serenity Prayer:

> *Grant me the serenity to accept the things I cannot change,*
> *the courage to change the things I can,*
> *and the wisdom to know the difference.*

Surrendering to Life is the serenity of accepting the things I cannot change—like the diagnosis of cancer. Now, do I have the courage to change my attitude and gaze at cancer with tenderness? Do I have the courage to invite it into my life and ask what it has to teach me? Do I have the courage to say *Namaste* to cancer?

Martial arts calls this attitude of surrender "bowing to life." My favorite verse from the *Tao Te Ching* says,

"Yield and overcome." I like this idea of bowing and yielding, because those images show me that I have to let go of something. And that's what Buddhism calls this surrendering to Life—"letting go." Letting go of my grasp, my desire to control things. Relinquishing my wanting, wanting things to be different than they are. It's the Third Noble Truth, usually called, simply, "cessation"—the ceasing of craving.

If I were a different person, maybe I could call it cooperating with Life or living harmoniously with Life, but strong-willed Cheryl does have to bow down and surrender. My ninety-three-year-old hospice client calls it "Not my will, but thine."* Letting go of my will has not been easy. I've spent way too much of my life spitting into the wind. It has not been in my nature to simply join with whatever's happening in the moment with full compliance.

You can call this act of surrender, this grace of surrender, whatever you want to. The Beatles sing "Let It Be."Tevye, in the *Fiddler on the Roof*, celebrates "*L'chaim.*" To life!

Zen refers to it as beginner's mind or don't-know mind. "In the expert's mind, there are few possibilities; in the beginner's mind, there are many." May I have the beginner's mind to see everything as new and fresh. May I surrender to the mind that does not know. Oh, that's such an uncomfortable state of mind—not knowing.

---

* Luke 22:42.

I may as well surrender to the river of life that is flowing through me. I may as well relax and go with the flow, not knowing where it will take me.

The Two Darts

WELCOME TO THE human body. Because we have a body, pain is inevitable. You can't have one without the other. Whether or not we suffer from that pain is our choice. Suffering is optional. The Buddha used the parable of the two darts to explain how this works: "It is as if a woman were pierced by a dart and, following the first piercing, she is hit by a second dart. So she will experience feelings caused by two darts: a bodily and a mental feeling."

The Buddha is using the example of physical pain, but usually what we are dealing with when we hear the word *cancer* is a heck of a lot of mental pain. *Oh, no. Not me! What am I going to do?* And then we stab ourselves again and again with a story about that original pain, the word *cancer*.

Shinzen Young elegantly sums up this *sutta* in a formula:

Pain × Resistance = Suffering

When we resist what is happening *(Oh, no! Why me? I don't want this!)*, we increase our suffering, our unease, our ill-at-easeness.

One possibility is to simply stick with the original pain, the first dart: the word *cancer*. Our minds don't really need to go any further than that. Our minds don't need to have an opinion or make up a story.

The Buddha goes on to say:

> But when a well-taught noble disciple is touched by a painful feeling, she will not worry nor grieve and lament, she will not beat her [cancerous] breast and weep, nor will she be distraught. It is *one* kind of feeling she experiences, a bodily one, but not a [subsequent] mental feeling. It is as if a woman were pierced by a dart, but was not hit by a second dart following the first one. So this person experiences feelings caused by a single dart only.
>
> Having been touched by that painful feeling, she does not resist (and resent) it. Hence, no underlying tendency of resistance against that painful feeling comes to underlie (her mind)."

I have received one dart: the word *cancer*. It's my choice whether or not to flagellate myself with that word and stick second darts all over my mind as if it were a voodoo doll.

I watch my friends unwittingly stick second darts into themselves. "Oh, no, Cheryl!" or "Oh, that's terrible!" or "Cancer is such a demon."

Before I heard the concept of the second dart, I

spent a year sticking second darts into my mind because I despised my supervisor at work. "Just drop it, Cheryl," my friends said. They were tired of hearing me complain. But I didn't know how to "just drop it."

I spent a decade of my life sticking darts into my heart because I was single and all my friends were married with children. I have wasted a lot of time beating my breast about what should or shouldn't happen, about how life should or shouldn't go.

Now I have the second-dart early-detection system—mindfulness of the mind. I can see and label the first dart and then watch various second darts try to pin themselves in my mind. Now I *can* "drop it" (maybe again and again), thanks to the teaching of the second dart.

Another Second Dart

THE DAY AFTER my diagnosis, I felt my first second dart of *I have cancer all over my body, and I don't know it*. I pulled out that second dart by using the inquiry process of The Work.* Just because I have a thought doesn't mean that it's true or that I have to believe it. When I believe my stressful thoughts, I suffer; when I don't believe them, I don't suffer. Happiness and fearlessness are nearby, if I can only clear away the clutter of the mind and notice them.

My mind has all the naïveté of a three-year-old who believes everything her mommy tells her. *If I think it, it must be true.* Question that thought.

Because I have a lot of experience recognizing second darts, I was able to notice those little buggers and sidestep most of them. But another second dart did land and lodge itself in my mind right after a friend gave me

---

* The Work consists of four questions and three turn-arounds. The questions are 1. Is it true? (Yes or no.) 2. Can you absolutely know that it's true? (Yes or no.) 3. How do you react, what happens when you believe that thought? 4. Who would you be without the thought? The three turn-arounds are three opposite thoughts to the original stressful thought.

some unwanted advice. *She should mind her own business.* *Harrumph.* I huffed out another breath. *She should mind her own business.* Oh-oh, that second dart was sticking itself more deeply, this time near my heart. It doesn't feel good to be mad at a friend.

She should mind her own business. Is that true?

Well, yes and no. She is expressing how much she cares for me, even if I don't like the way she is doing it. Since I have to answer *yes* or *no*, the answer is no.

Now, for the turnarounds. Turning around the original stressful thought, writing down its opposites, often reveals something about myself.

I should mind my own business.

Well, duh. Yes, I should mind my own business, and get my nose out of her business. Right now. I have plenty of business of my own to pay attention to.

She shouldn't mind her own business.

Since she's had breast cancer recently, she might have some good ideas for me. And she's a friend. This is what friends do—they dare to make my business their business. I often do this myself.

I should mind her own business.

When she shares something personal with me, I should pay attention and be more mindful of her feelings. Sometimes I'm a bit cavalier with someone else's tender feelings.

Her business should mind me.

This should (re)mind me to stick to my own business.

One of these turnarounds really got to me, and that was to be more mindful of her feelings when she shares something personal. Here I am asking her to be more mindful of my feelings, when, actually, *I'm* the one who needs to be more mindful of *her* feelings.

Oh, the mind is so tricky. This is just another example of how it projects its own bad habits onto someone else, while it looks the other way and whistles, "Who? Me? No! Not me. I'm innocent." Ha!

Like when I go out to the car, and the key isn't in it. *Bill!* I think, and begin to simmer. Then I find the key in my own coat pocket. That is projection.

The mind pretends to be minding its own business right after it's pinned its little secret on someone else. Then it pouts, *Ouch! My feelings are hurt.* Or the mind is irritated. *Why can't they just . . . ?*

Oh, it feels so good to write the mind down on paper. It's the only way I can pin it down.

No Second Opinion

MICHELLE, WHO HAD breast cancer ten years ago, thought I really should go to the big city to get a second opinion about my diagnosis and treatment. I had enough confidence in our local medical services to decide to stay small-town.

Here's how "big-city" looked to me. First, I would have to call the big, important cancer center and make an appointment. With whom? That would take time and many more phone calls to figure out. I'm not really good about making phone calls; I avoid them if at all possible.

I would have to drive two hours to the city and then drive in the city for another half hour. Find a place to park. Pay through the wazoo to park my car. Not know where I am going. Find where I am going. Wait.

Even though I would have my medical records sent to the city hospital, what do you want to bet that some piece of information would be missing? Or that I would have to wait or be sent for testing?

This second opinion would take not only an entire day, it would take a previous day's worth of hours to arrange everything.

I'm just not that afraid. I'm not fearful enough to

want to twist my panties (or bra) into that knot. I'm confident about our local services. I have no doubts. I can stay local, drive twenty minutes to the hospital, be done in an hour, and drive home. So much less stress.

Certainly, there are times for second opinions. When the body gets complicated, or when it has a rare ailment and the specialty clinic is in the big city. These are the times when it makes sense to go to the experts. I understood that my cancer was small and run-of-the-mill. If that wasn't correct, I would find out soon enough.

One friend of a friend went to Sloan-Kettering in New York City for her cancer treatment. Among other things, they recommended green tea extract and a mushroom supplement—both of which are available at my local holistic health center. Dana Farber Cancer Institute in Boston offers acupuncture for those undergoing radiation. I don't need to drive to Boston for that treatment.

A nurse tells me there are regional differences in cancer treatments. My region includes the nearest big city. I wasn't sure that my treatment in the big city would be much different from what I could obtain locally. It sounds to me as though every cancer care provider has a recipe book, a flowchart for if-this-then-that. I have drawn many flowcharts in my several computer programming classes. I can easily imagine an entire map of treatment options, depending on many variables.

The advantage in a small town is that people know each other, and word travels if something goes wrong. I had heard that my surgeon's wife had breast cancer three years ago, and that in itself recommended him to me. (He also went to summer camp with my neighbor's brother when he was twelve.) Dr. Rosen had a plaque on his desk from the American Cancer Society "for outstanding service to the cause of cancer control."

As Americans, we believe strongly in freedom of choice. Yet sometimes we feel overwhelmed by all the choices, all the possibilities we have at our fingertips or within a two-hour drive from home. We rake the choices over and over in our minds, believing that one of them will be "best" (as if that is true). At the same time, we disbelieve our own powers of prognostication. *Which one? Which one? This one? Or that one?* (Worry, worry.)

Sometimes it's better to have fewer choices.

Sometimes small is beautiful, and small-town feels very beautiful indeed, especially when it's conducive to a beautiful, stress-free mind.

MRI

A WEEK BEFORE MY surgery, I went in for a breast MRI. I'd been in an MRI twice before, both times for studies of meditators. The first time, I was at the Yale–New Haven hospital and inside the MRI for two hours, meditating for a few minutes, then hearing instructions for the next meditation. After lying absolutely still for so long and meditating, even though in short bursts, I entered an altered state. Through my headphone/earmuffs the jackhammering of the magnets started to sound like crickets. I felt totally blissed out.

As Shinzen Young says, "The longer we sit, the deeper we go." I was certainly feeling that the longer I lay there, meditating in the MRI, the deeper I went.

Several friends who have had MRIs have reported claustrophobia, twitchiness, and inability to tolerate the extremely loud banging—although one friend quipped, "I always have liked banging."

Friends offered all sorts of helpful advice. Wear earplugs. Take your own music because you don't want to be at the mercy of hospital Muzak. One friend had to listen to "Manic Monday" during her MRI, not the sort of thing you would choose for yourself.

For the breast MRI, I lay face down with my arms stretched above me, while my breasts were hanging down through an opening in the bed.

Knowing I'd have to hold this position for twenty minutes, I tried to make sure I was as comfortable as possible to start with. This is one example of how meditation comes in handy—being able to bear a slightly awkward position for a little while, and stay still, even when it becomes a bit uncomfortable.

I knew that the MRI was important to the surgeon; it would give him an additional image to "look" at the cancer on my chest wall; it would allow him to assess his plan for my lumpectomy. He would be able to see if there was an undetected cancer in my other breast, or if one of my lymph nodes was abnormally large and therefore possibly infected with cancer. It takes a few days for the MRI to be "read" and a report written, so the surgeon would have the information seven days hence.

More than anything, I wanted the surgery to proceed on schedule, and I was doing everything in my power to jump through all the required hoops. If this meant lying still, face down, for twenty minutes, I would do it.

As the bed moved into the tunnel, I relaxed and began to meditate, noticing my breath, noticing the clanging, noticing the half-second of calm between the clangs, noticing that despite the small discomfort, I was actually all right.

Maybe I should just be listening to Bob Marley.

"Don't worry about a thing, 'cause every little thing is gonna be all right."

Just as in meditation, the position became slightly uncomfortable—my left arm wanted to move. I recalled my intention, just as I do in meditation. I breathed into the slight ache, and, on the outbreath, made a conscious effort to relax. I remembered a teaching by the Vietnamese monk Thich Nhat Hanh: "Breathing in, I calm body and mind. Breathing out, I smile." When I focused on these words, the ache receded, the clanging receded, and then it stopped.

"Okay," the technician said, and I smiled.

My Legacy #1

I N THE DAYS after receiving my diagnosis but before surgery, in that never-never land of not knowing, in the limbo of uncertainty, I dug out my annual writing booklets and books. I've been writing these since 2002. For the first seven years, I spent hours at Lotus Graphics each November photocopying them—a different color of paper for each section—and then having these booklets spiral bound. That was the beginning of my self-publishing. A very small run, I might add.

When I became an official publisher in 2010, I had my annual books printed-on-demand at Lightning Source. Now that I knew a book designer who could, for not much money, create a beautiful cover and lay out the pages, publishing a "real" book turned out to be pretty easy. At first, I said, "I know this looks like a real book," as I handed a copy to a friend, before adding, "but it's not."

Oh, the many ways in which we women discount ourselves. I've stopped dissing myself. Now I smile when someone exclaims, "Oh, you have another book!" What I have is another immortality project. But my readers report that they enjoy this taste of ordinary life, and they always chuckle at the further adventures of that character

Bill. Some of my memoir pieces make certain readers cringe, which I think is the best review I've ever received.

Looking back at those earlier Lotus Graphics–produced booklets, I was wondering if I should make the effort to have those officially published, too, so that they look like real books. The advantage of using Lightning Source is that the books automatically show up on Amazon as well as the computer screens of every bookstore in the country. So far, each one of my books has been selling about five copies a year.

By contemplating this question, I was really asking myself, *What do I want to leave behind? What is my legacy? How do I want to be remembered?* But also, and perhaps more importantly, *What is my purpose in life?*

Since 2010 I've hired a real editor for my annual book, with the result that my writing has improved bit by bit, here and there. Going back to the earlier books would mean a hefty editing project. And how would that read, with this year's editing on top of ten-year-old writing?

Is this impulse to officially print my old booklets just my ego talking? (Well, yes, of course it is. The "I" wants to be remembered.) Or is it a gentle nudge from Life whispering in my ear, "Go ahead. Do it. Do it now. Later may be too late."

I've heard enough stories of a person's life work being thrown out in the trash at her death—crafts she has made, research she has done, or books she has written. Van Gogh's mother threw away crates of his paintings, so I can predict that my life's work will go straight into the dumpster, too. Until then, I'll write and publish—on my blog, on Facebook, and once a year in a book of reflections.

Originally, I wanted my writing to send a message-in-a-bottle to future generations of my family, even though they won't be interested in my stories until after I am dead. But it turns out that my audience is my own generation—people who nod their heads while reading one of my essays, people who call my Facebook posts "thought pokers." My writing turns out to be here and now; this is my actual legacy, my purpose, every day that my blog appears on Facebook. Here. And gone from the reader's consciousness in an instant—yet making even that slight impression, that gentle reminder of the Dharma, is sufficient for my heart and mind. Part of my intention is to inspire people to live in accord with their hearts.

Shall I republish my older collections for a wider audience? What is my legacy, really?

Three years ago, I divided those annual collections into six themed e-books. That project fell off my radar screen after four of them were edited. There they sit in my computer, like a half-finished quilt or a half-done painting.

Life is drawing my attention to them, like dust bunnies in the corner. *Clean out your files. Clean up your act. If you don't do it, no one else will.* Do it yourself, and do it *for* yourself. I recall and recommit to my life's purpose.

Thirty years ago, I committed to writing. At first, of

course, I felt tentative about it. After a few years, one friend said, "You sure do write a lot," as if I wrote too much. I wondered whether I should stop writing, but then I decided that part of my purpose of being on this earth (as confirmed, incidentally, by my astrology chart) was to write. It doesn't matter whether my writing is "good" (I'm sure it does not meet the high standards of some writerly friends); my writing is good enough.

Now that I am looking the Heavenly Messengers square in the eye, it is time to remember the purpose of my life and act accordingly, even if no one remembers me. (I know from my own experience how quickly deceased friends fall off my radar screen.) I need to live my purpose for myself. That is my real legacy—to be the most true and most authentic Cheryl Wilfong that I can be.

Contentment

I N THE SUMMER and fall, I love to take my kayak
to the river in the early evening. Often, I simply push
out from shore, paddle a few strokes, and rest in the flow
of the river. My 70-percent-water body tunes in to the
gently flowing river. I feel at rest, at one with the river.
Nowhere to go and nothing to do. Contentment.

The phone and the watch have been left behind.
Now it is only me and the river. I let it take me where
it will. Often, I float downstream with the current, but
sometimes, mysteriously, it takes me upstream. I do not
exert my will. I go where I am sent. Contentment.

When I put worry, fear, and anxiety on hold, I have
a chance of accepting life just as it is without resistance,
without arguing with Life. As Byron Katie says, "When
you argue with reality, you lose. But only 100 percent of
the time."

Oh, I've argued with life, plenty. Wanting relationships after they have ended. Wishing that troublesome
people would disappear from my life. All that resisting
reality does is to blur my vision so that I don't see what's
right in front of my nose. If I can hold my horses for a
minute, if I can simply push the pause button on the

stories my mind is telling itself, then I can begin to see things just as they are.

When I accept things as they really are, I experience a moment of wishlessness—not wishing for things to be different. This state of wishlessness feels like contentment in the body. I allow things to be just as they are. The river of life flows on, and I am floating with it.

Fine

I USED TO TALK to my dad on the phone every Sunday afternoon. When I asked him how he was, even in the last years of his life, when he was constantly chilly from kidney failure, he always answered: "Fine." Even in the days before he died, at age seventy-nine, in 1997, he was "fine."

After those phone calls with Dad, I would talk to my brother Beau, who lived next door to Dad and worked for him as his general manager. "Dad had a colonoscopy and they removed a polyp the size of a turkey egg." "Dad's BUN levels are going up." "His kidneys are functioning at 25 percent." Then "15 percent." Then "He's having a stent installed in his abdomen so he can do his own dialysis exchanges."

Still, during every Sunday phone call, Dad would say he was "fine." I chalked it up to his Christian Science upbringing. No negative thinking. He was a mind-over-matter man. And his company was called Fine Builders.

When I visited him in Indiana every three months, he would recommend something to me—New Balance shoes or a Waterpik or an electric toothbrush. I didn't put two and two together. He was recommending these things to me because his doctor or dentist had recommended them to him.

Twenty years later, I see that Dad was giving me a spiritual teaching, even though he was not a spiritual man.

Now that New Balance shoes (with orthotics), a Waterpik, and an electric toothbrush are part of my daily life, I too consider myself to be "fine." Now that I have a diagnosis of breast cancer, I actually feel fine. And, more importantly, my thinking is "fine." Thanks to the inquiry process of The Work, I can question each stressful thought as it comes up and set it loose, leaving me in the present moment of a warm house on a snowy day.

I could worry about the doctor's appointment tomorrow, but why bother? Worry is a useless waste of energy. Today I can't know what isn't known to me, so why fret?

I was at the hospital twice last week having five different tests. It was easy. It was quick. It was fine.

And three days before surgery, so am I.

Divine Love

I SAY THAT MY dad wasn't a spiritual man, yet every evening at the dinner table he said grace. "Divine Love always has met, and always will meet every human need. Give us grace for today, and feed the family to perfection."

I had no idea that this was a Christian Science blessing, nor that he had mangled the last line, which should be "feed the famished affections." I never took the blessing to heart, nor even gave it a second thought. It was just something Dad did. Like his insistence that we all eat dinner together. When Mom said, "Dinner's ready," we were all sitting at our places within a minute. Dad did not tolerate lateness. No excuses, not even sickness.

I suppose that Dad had heard his own father say this grace. Maybe it was his father who had transformed the last line. "Feed the family to perfection" makes a lot more sense if you're at the head of a table of ten children during the Great Depression. And since that little house had only two rooms, the dinner table was on the back porch, with a bench that was hinged onto the wall of the house. Every meal was a picnic, even in the winter.

For his own family, Dad soon changed the last phrase to his own liking, since we always had more than enough on our own dinner table. "Give us grace for today, and feed the hungry and needy." He had been hungry as a child; he had been needy.

"Divine Love always has met and always will meet every human need," wrote Mary Baker Eddy. Although *Science and Health* is difficult to decipher, I suspect that she was an awakened woman, though constrained by nineteenth-century language and beliefs. How does anyone fit the unsayable into the prevailing norms of those days? Even Ralph Waldo Emerson and the Transcendentalists, with whom I resonated as a junior in high school, are a slog to actually sit down and read. Just pass me the cherry-picked excerpts.

As I contemplate "Divine Love always has met and always will meet every human need," I begin to hear my own rephrasing. *I surrender to Life.* Trusting that Life will meet my needs. Not necessarily the needs that I think I have, though that often happens too. Trusting that Life will meet the needs I didn't even know I had.

Give me the grace to trust Life as it unfolds, to trust "Divine Love," if that's what you want to call it. Give me the grace to feed my famished mind, the mind that constantly feels something is missing, something is lacking, the mind that worries about the uncertainties of life, the mind that wants something other than what is.

What's missing is certainty and stability. The Buddha calls this transience or impermanence one of the three characteristics of all experience. Uncertainty is always standing on the sidelines of our daily life, but we try not to notice it in favor of the known, the certain, and what we think we can control.

In fact, I don't know what's going to happen next. If I look closely, I never actually know what's going to happen next. Not really, though usually I have a pretty good guess. But now, in the midst of a cancer diagnosis, the mind begins to juggle one unknown after another, and begins to feel desperate. Mary Baker Eddy's word is "famished." The mind is starving for certainty.

How can I hold this hunger to know? By feeding my mind "affection," kindness, and benevolence. Trusting that the world is a friendly place. Can I feed "affection," can I offer acceptance to my own and to those famished minds, all of our minds that hunger for something that is missing?

Prayer

IF YOU ASKED me, I would say I don't know a thing about prayer. I suppose that's because, when I was sixteen, I off-loaded prayer along with going to church and believing in God, and I never looked back.

A sister breast-cancer survivor recommended Anne Lamott's book on prayer: *Help, Thanks, Wow: The Three Essential Prayers*. When you put it that way, I suspect we all know more about prayer than we may think we do. Prayer isn't always just a call for help, though distress is often the warning signal that drives us onto a spiritual path.

When life takes a turn that we did not expect and that we do not want, we suddenly feel out of our depth. *Help! Help me!* Though some Christian friends feel a need to address this request to *someone*, I do not. I've always been a self-reliant, self-help type of gal—even after I glimpsed that there is no self to help.

When our friends are in need of help, our hearts naturally open to their suffering. This is called compassion. When we ourselves are in distress, we can practice self-compassion.

If I look closely, I find that I do have some very

simple prayers. After all, some prayers are formulas, to be repeated over and over. Some examples of "prayers" for compassion are *May you be free from suffering* or *May I be held in compassion.*

Place your hand on your heart. Now. Breathe. Breathe in your suffering, your heartache. Perhaps it feels dark and heavy. Breathe out light and caring. The heart is a marvelous transformer. The heart has the power to change your mind. Spend a few minutes sinking into receiving the pain (your own or that of another). *Ouch! It hurts.* Really soak into it, using mindfulness like acupressure on that tender spot. Feel the tenderness of the pain, and feel tender toward yourself. Then, as you breathe out light, practice giving care (to yourself or another). This might be a wordless prayer, or you might augment it with words of compassion.

I've come up with my own compassion prayer, what I call "caring and bearing." I care, and I can bear feeling the other person's suffering—or my own—without a need to change anything. For self-compassion, I paraphrase T. S. Eliot: *Teach me to care and not to care.* This conundrum, this paradox, this bothness of seeming opposites has the power to stop my mind and expand my heart. Caring and not caring calls for radical acceptance of what is. It calls us out of the rational world of this-or-that and into the inexplicable sacredness of the allness of life.

Sometimes I call to mind the image of an eight-foot-tall Kuan Yin I saw in a Chinese temple in Honolulu. That Kuan Yin was no spring chicken; she had jowls. She was a woman who had seen a lot of life. Tears came to my eyes as I gazed at her—a woman who has seen everything life can dish out and who still cares, deeply.

Loving-kindness, or *metta*, is another prayer. *May I feel safe. May I feel happy. May I feel healthy. May I feel peaceful. In the midst of this situation, may I feel safe.*

We begin with ourselves and gradually expand our circle of kindness to loved ones (easy), friends (easy), our community (okay), neutral people (them? but I don't even know their names), and finally, a difficult person (gulp). The word *kindness* is related to the word *kin*. When we practice kindness, we practice feeling kinship with other beings. I try to simply feel these well wishes in my heart and turn them loose. Sometimes (but not always) they infuse my body. Ahhh. Delicious. So *this* is what an open heart feels like.

We practice loving-kindness as an expression of our caring, our kindness toward all living beings. Even though *metta* doesn't sound so much like a prayer for help, the original intent of *metta* was to free people from fear. The direct translation of the words the Buddha spoke is this: *May I be free from affliction. May I be free from ill will. May I be free from anxiety. And may I maintain well-being in myself.*

In the West, the phrases for *metta* are seldom called prayers, but my friend Khin in Burma tells me she prays for me every day. By this I know she means she is sending me the well-wishes of loving-kindness.

Sometimes I get creative and send *metta* to an irritating situation. For instance, once I was annoyed by the new furnace in the room next to the meditation hall. In my imagination, I offered the furnace loads of flowers for keeping the hall warm. When I returned to another retreat a year later, I barely noticed the furnace purring on and off, on and off.

Feel free to send *metta* toward any*thing* as well as any*one* you have a grudge against. Don't start with your worst enemy—which might be cancer. Start with something easier.

Sometimes the help we need (but don't necessarily want) is acceptance of the situation in which we find ourselves. My favorite prayer for equanimity is: *May I accept things as they are. May I see and accept things as they really are.* This is the place where we invite help of a different sort: help move my ego out of the way. This is the long out-breath when we say "Not my will, but thine." Or as A.A. says, "Let go and let God." The Serenity Prayer is another equanimity prayer.

Compassion, loving-kindness, and equanimity are three of the four divine abodes. All these immeasurable, boundless qualities have traditional "prayers" or phrases associated with them. One way to view prayer is as a connection to the divine. With the divine abodes, we seek to connect with our own divine emotions, the divine that naturally lives in our very own hearts.

The fourth divine abode is appreciative joy, which can start with your own personal prayer of gratitude. This is an example of the *Thanks* prayer that Anne Lamott talks about.

Brother David Steindl-Rast describes the difference

between thankfulness and gratefulness.* Thankfulness requires someone or something to give thanks to. Gratitude is the moment before thankfulness when you simply *feel* blessed or wholeheartedly grateful.

The practice of gratitude begins with listing a few gratitudes. You then sink into feeling one of them. Wallow around in this blessing for thirty seconds. (Even though the mind wanders away, keep coming back to this one gratitude.) Spending thirty seconds rewires your neural networks so that, eventually, gratitude becomes a habit. When you drink in gratitude for twenty or thirty seconds, the heart opens. That flicker of *ahhh* is a prayer. That evanescent feeling of joy, whether you've created it or it has simply arrived, is the *Wow* prayer that Anne Lamott refers to.

Wow! I have running water. And electricity. Wow! I feel safe in my house. Wow! I'm a woman who can drive a car (there are countries where women cannot drive), and I can even feel safe at night driving by myself. Or, double wow, I feel safe walking in the dark by myself. These things that we take for granted are truly amazing when you stop to think about them.

Mary Oliver writes in her poem "When Death Comes,"

> *When it's over, I want to say: all my life*
> *I was a bride married to amazement.*

---

* See: gratefulness.org.

Mary Oliver writes many amazement poems. If your mind feels stuck, and you can't grow any amazement today, read a Mary Oliver poem to jump-start your own *Wow* prayer.

Another kind of prayer is listening to the sounds of silence. In fact, the mind doesn't need to be silent to hear the sound of silence. We can notice the silence between thoughts or the silence behind the chattering mind.

I often tell a story at the beginning of an introductory meditation class to a multi-faith group. When Dan Rather was interviewing Mother Teresa in 1986, he asked her what she said when she prayed. "Oh, I don't say anything," she said. "I listen."

"Well then, what does God say?" Dan Rather asked.

"Oh," said Mother Teresa, "He doesn't say anything. He's listening, too."

Christians call the sound of silence "communion with God." I call it "resting on the ocean of Life." Meditators call it "open awareness." This is an excellent place to ask "Who am I?" or "Who is meditating?" or "Who is walking?"—and notice the silent answer.

My prayers often take the form of self-talk to bolster my wholesome intentions when my puppy mind wants to chew on the same old raggedy thought again. *I can't know what I don't know.* Or I tell myself: *It's useless to worry.* Or I give myself a pep talk: *Surrender to Life. Life has been good to me so far.* Or I remind myself: *When I argue with reality, I always lose.*

Surprisingly, I circle back to the grace my father said

every night at the dinner table fifty years ago. *Divine Love always has met and always will meet every human need.* Whenever something goes awry, I trot out this little prayer to feel whether I can believe it, whether I can fall into that Divine Love that knows better than I do exactly what this human needs in this frustrating or unwanted situation.

"Cheryl, You Should Be More Worried"

MARIA, WHO HAD breast cancer a few years ago, told me, "Cheryl, you should be worried." Maria was quite concerned that I was not worried.

I was at a loss as to how to respond to her, so I simply nodded. Not a nod of agreement, but a nod to say, *I hear you.*

I couldn't think of a single reason why I should cultivate worry or the habit of worry. I felt fine without it. Worry is a stressor. Worry is a misuse of imagination. Worry is called a hindrance to the spiritual path because it distracts our minds from meditation. Worry obscures our tender hearts.

I suspect Maria thought that worry would motivate me to *do* something in the ten days between diagnosis and my scheduled surgery. I seemed to be just passively accepting the services offered at Brattleboro Memorial Hospital when I could be doing so much more. To me, "doing so much more" sounded so much more stressful.

Perhaps Maria thought worrying would help me protect my health. If I worried, I would be more vigilant.

I'd spend more time reading more books, asking more questions, putting cancer at the center of my life. Instead of reading books I was writing books, living my life, editing one manuscript, publishing another, writing another one. I was just living my ordinary life as if I didn't understand the word *cancer* as a giant blinking red light in the middle of my life, warning me to drop everything and focus on it. As if I didn't understand that cancer was *bad*.

Worry might also be helpful for planning my treatment. Of course, the treatment wouldn't happen for two more months, but I should start planning now, for God's sake.

There I was, living one day at a time, as if that's an actual way to live. How exasperating for my dear friend!

I had been meditating for years, pulling the supporting pins out from that belief in a future. The future is an idea we have; it's a thought. And then we believe it. And all the time, we are right here in the present moment, the only place our body-minds can ever be. Our thought of a future is happening right now. Worry depends on (1) believing there is a future, and (2) believing that something bad is going to happen in that future.

"Bad" is an idea that depends on there being a "good." But what if there's only Life happening? In one sense, the "bad" had already happened—a diagnosis of cancer. (And even there, I could make a case for the diagnosis being a good thing. Now that the cancer had been discovered, I was doing something about it.) What other "bad" thing might lie in my (nonexistent) future? More cancer? Death? Death lies in all of our futures.

Death is bad only for the ego. No self, no problem. I'd been practicing dying to the ego, moment by moment, for years. Oh, sure, my ego still shows up on a daily basis, but I do have moments of Life simply flowing through me, when my sense of self mysteriously floats away for a few seconds or a few minutes.

In those few moments of not-self, there are no worries and no fear. Only happiness.

I asked Maria if she was afraid. "Oh, no," she said. "Not me. Not at all."

Resilience

"**Y**OU ARE SO resilient, Cheryl," says Bill, shaking his head, because he is not. He's just given me a piece of bad news about repairs to our truck, which he's been mulling over all afternoon.

"Oh, Bill," I say, "Don't worry. We can . . ." and I proceed to give him three possible options. I'm not sure if any of the three options will actually work out; only time will tell.

Neuroscientists have developed scales for six qualities that are measurable in the brain—resilience, outlook, self-awareness, attention, social intuition, and sensitivity to context. I happen to have fairly high resilience and an optimistic outlook. Therapy in my thirties moved my self-awareness from near zero to above average. My attention is above average, but not really focused enough to attain meditative states of concentration. My social intuition is below average; I just don't pick up as many conversational cues as Bill does. And my sensitivity to context, well, you might judge me as being a bit blunt because I write about things that would embarrass someone else.

My natural resilience helps me a lot in this diagnosis and treatment of cancer.

Being "too" high in resilience, being too fast to recover from setbacks, can make my friends think that I am unemotional, walled off, or uncaring. It's as if a hard ball has just bounced off my internal trampoline without leaving a bruise. To someone who is less resilient, for whom the hard ball lands hard, my response to their difficult situation can feel unempathic. If they are sympathizing with me, my too-resilient response can make them feel that I've short-circuited them when I say, "Oh, I feel fine," leaving them with tender feelings that I've just overridden (due to my lower sensitivity to context).

The first step to developing greater resilience is mindfulness, because mindfulness keeps me closer to the present moment and less likely to wallow in setbacks of the past or to catastrophize about the future.

Resilience is one place where my natural problem-solving ability comes in handy. I can "see" the steps to take in order to head toward a positive solution to adversity, like making lemonade out of lemons.

Reframing is also an excellent way to develop resilience. Reframing means looking at the same situation from a different and more positive angle. I became acquainted with reframing when I was a psychotherapist, practicing it often with my clients.

I teach meditation at a nearby county jail, on the women's block. Recently, I told one prisoner-meditator at the jail, who always wears white instead of regulation orange, that people on retreat in Asia and India wear white. She has now, on her own, reframed her jail experience as a nine-month retreat.

In the past several years, I've become more adept at reframing through doing the inquiry process of The Work. Coming up with three turnarounds for any stressful thought, and seeing how these three opposite thoughts can be equally true (and sometimes truer than the original stressful thought) erodes the stressor thought and washes it away. Then letting go just naturally happens. I don't let go of the stressful thought; the stressful thought lets go of me.

I've also watched my teacher, Shinzen Young, respond to questions from meditation students. I have never heard him say or even imply that anyone is wrong; he simply reframes it. "It's all good," he says.

My own meditation students often want to make themselves wrong or bad. *Oh, I'm not a good meditator. I don't know how. . . . I can't still my mind.* (Of course you can't!) Whatever they say, I simply reframe it by pointing out the positive in what they perceive as negative. A yoga teacher who was taking my Introduction to Insight Meditation course finally said to me, "I can't do anything wrong in this class." That made me smile.

In mindfulness meditation, we are practicing, practicing nonjudgmental awareness. Not judging our experience or anyone else's. Mindfulness and suspension of judgment add up to resilience. Here and now.

Overly Optimistic

A FEW FRIENDS FELT I was being overly optimistic about my diagnosis. Carla thought I should be taking this word *cancer* much more seriously than I seemed to be doing. She thought I should pull out all the stops. Go to Dana Farber in Boston. Get a second opinion. I should read more books. Above all, I should be going to a support group to help me deal with my feelings.

Yet I had stopped. I stopped my mind from worrying every time I caught it sneaking into the future, and I stopped my cancer shopping in Brattleboro. I was buying local—at Brattleboro Memorial Hospital.

The problem with being overly optimistic is that my friends had nowhere to put their own feelings of fear and worry. It would have been so much easier if I had just settled down and been a problem that they, in their wisdom, could fix. But I wasn't cooperating. I didn't feel I had a problem. I had breast cancer, and then it was removed. The rest is just a story. Oh, how we love our stories, because who would we be without them? Without our stories of our selves, we are face to face with the Buddha's most difficult teaching: not-self.

I went to a personal growth workshop where one

of the exercises was to write our most stressful story as a newspaper article. "Just the facts, ma'am." *Woman Diagnosed with Breast Cancer to Have Lumpectomy. After surgery, she will have a month of healing at home followed by recommended treatment.* Those are the facts, and that's really all there is. Everything else is story, the mind trying to make sense of a torrent of emotion. You can see that a personal story full of ups and downs, suspense and unexpected turns, greed and revenge, lust and jealousy is much more interesting and attention-getting than the factual, bare-bones report. A story is stressful.

When I write my story in the third person, as if it is happening to someone else, I see that "my" story is not personal. Millions of other women with breast cancer have a similar story. My emotions are very personal, of course, because breast cancer is happening to *me*.

If my ego were miraculously removed, if my ego could float away for even a moment, I would see that this story, "my" story, is simply life unfolding, a body aging with a disease. However, the disease of my body does not have to cause dis-ease in my mind.

Our minds naturally have a negativity bias. We want to know the bad news. We focus on the worst-case scenario. As one neuroscientist says, "Our minds are like Velcro for the negative and Teflon for the positive." The negative makes a much more riveting story.

My practice—you can call it optimistic, if you wish—is to accentuate the positive by focusing on all the good things that are happening. It's so good to have a knowledgeable surgeon, an efficient hospital, a caring nurse navigator, a helpful radiologist, and friends. All so good. And I feel so grateful.

Am I being naive? My intention is to be positive, not to be a Pollyanna. A Pollyanna is fake positivity. Pollyanna is another word for "spiritual bypass"—plastering over dark feelings with a veneer of "nice." A spiritual bypass means looking good, perhaps even oh-so-spiritual, to other people, while a tangle of torment—worry and fear—is locked in the subbasement of the mind. A spiritual bypass means pretending to be something or someone I am not. But I've never been good at veneer; veneer feels false.

By looking on the bright side, I am taking my Dharma friend Rick Hanson's advice.* I challenge myself to feel grateful for one thing for thirty seconds. That's how long it takes for neural networks to begin to rewire themselves in the body.

I start with the easy ones—like the radiologist who walked me to the surgeon's office and made my appointment for me. My heart melts at his kindness. My friend Barbara. My neighbors in my morning meditation group. Sink into gratitude. Savor it. Drink it in. Marinate in it. Once you start reviewing your life, you find blessings everywhere. *Hey! I'm alive!*

---

* Rick Hanson is the author of *Buddha's Brain: The Practical Neuroscience of Happiness, Love, and Wisdom* and *Hardwiring Happiness: The New Brain Science of Contentment, Calm, and Confidence.*

A few years ago, I practiced gratitude for two hours while I was having gum surgery. Grateful for eighteen shots of Novocain. Oh, yes! Grateful for the periodontist's training. Grateful for modern technology. My grandmother had all her teeth pulled at fifty-five, but when I was that age I still had all my teeth. And I could afford to pay for them. Grateful, grateful, grateful.

Our positivity becomes authentic and not sugarcoated when it is based on self-love rather than self-hatred. Self-hatred says or thinks "I'm so bad," but of course I don't want other people to see this, so I pretend to be nice.

Self-love is tender toward those jagged edges of my inner landscape. I love myself as I am—even when I'm feeling rotten, confused, and even hateful. Although self-love sounds selfish, it's like putting on your own oxygen mask first. Self-love follows the conventional wisdom that says, "You can't love anyone else if you don't love yourself."

I have so much to be grateful for. Life is actually meeting all my needs. You can call that optimistic or overly optimistic. One thing is for sure—it's a lot less stressful than its opposite.

T Minus 2 and Counting

TWO DAYS BEFORE surgery, I have another appointment to see the surgeon. Barbara comes with me. As Dr. Rosen talks, she takes notes in neat, legible handwriting. Having worked in outpatient surgery, she speaks medical lingo with the doc. As soon as she tells him what her experience was, I can see him relax, treating her as a colleague who understands everything he is saying.

She asks the surgeon clarifying questions, using the right jargon; the doctor looks at her, not at her ailing friend.

After the appointment, while Barbara and I are having tea in the hospital cafeteria, we review what we each heard. Today, there are no more decisions to make—we are receiving information about pre-surgery, surgery, and post-surgery. Mostly, I feel glad that things are going as planned.

She asks whether I want her to come to my surgery, but I think I can manage without her. Bill will go with me, and I'll ask a couple of other friends. Since she lives forty minutes away, today's appointment has taken her entire morning.

Even though Barbara is retired, she's busy cleaning up local rivers and conserving wildflowers. She spent many years on the conservation committee for the bedroom community of Swanzey, New Hampshire, which keeps building yet another big-box store on yet another marsh. She has a lot of conservation work to do. I feel extremely grateful that conserving my health is part of her service to the world around her.

Nurse Navigator

WHEN I HAD my second appointment with the surgeon, two days before surgery, he went to talk to the radiologist to find the answer to some question he had. While I was waiting, I hung out in a lounge near the mammography department. A few minutes later, a short woman walked in from the nearby stairwell. She came right over and said, "Hi. I'm Kelly McCue. I'm the Nurse Navigator."

"Hi," I said. "I'm Cheryl Wilfong." Somehow, I felt she already knew who I was.

"Yes," she said. "I read your blog this morning."

This is what I love about a small town.

"And I just read about you," I said, "in *Views of Dummerston*." *Views of Dummerston* is our town's quarterly newsletter, produced entirely by volunteers. It had just arrived in our mailbox the day before. "Congratulations, Kelly, on your PhD."

"Come into my office," Nurse Navigator Kelly said, and I followed her a few steps into a big room. She closed the door behind us.

"Here," she said, casting an eye over me. "Here's your cancer swag bag." From a wide cabinet with many shelves, she surveyed a foot-tall pile of handmade grocery-shopping bags, and chose a small bag in blue, turquoise, and green with green cloth handles.

"Here's a little tube of lidocaine," she said, reaching into her large cabinet and dropping a little tube into my attractive new swag bag that coordinated perfectly with my teal shirt and chartreuse down vest.

"And a tongue depressor." She added it to the swag bag while she continued talking. "Tomorrow you'll apply the lidocaine around your right nipple. It's your right breast, isn't it?" I nodded. "Apply the lidocaine about two hours before you come in to have the nuclear medicine injected. Then wrap the nipple with Saran Wrap so it will stay in place and won't stain your bra. What size bra do you wear?"

"Oh, gee, I don't know," I said. "I haven't worn a bra for forty years. 34B?"

"Here's some Chapstick, too," she said, reaching into a box on another shelf in the cabinet. I could see all colors of hand-knit caps, probably for those going through chemotherapy. Piles of turbans. A pile of hand-knit shawls. On a high shelf behind me stood a dozen mannequin heads wearing wigs. I could see that Kelly was your one-stop shopping center for all things related to cancer surgery and treatment. "Do you have any questions?" she asked.

"Well, Dr. Rosen is going on vacation on Saturday, but Pathology won't know whether or not my margins are clear until Tuesday. How can I find out the results?"

"Come in and see me," Kelly said. "I can tell you, because I have access to your medical records. I'm like a free doctor's appointment."

I was really liking Kelly, a no-nonsense woman who at the same time was kind and thoughtful. She covered all the bases.

"Here's my card," she said. "You can call or e-mail me anytime. I work Monday through Thursday."

Although I didn't have any more questions at the moment, I could see how Nurse Navigator Kelly could help a woman in distress. The NN has to be a Jane-of-all-trades, able to fill gaps resulting from vacations or short-sightedness, and able to respond to any emergency. She was the safety net for the entire oncology department.

Even though I had spent only five minutes with Kelly, I already felt that she was a friend, and that I could ask her *anything*. I felt so grateful to her and to the little Brattleboro Memorial Hospital for providing such continuity of service and care, and caring.

What's Your Fear Level?

"WHAT'S YOUR FEAR level?" my friend, the rabbi asked.

I hesitated for a split second. I wanted to say zero, but maybe I should say "one"? Would I be bragging if I said "zero"? Was fear hiding somewhere and I simply wasn't recognizing it? But "one" didn't feel honest.

"Zero," I said.

I have breast cancer. I've known this for ten days. I'm having a lumpectomy tomorrow. Today, nuclear isotopes will be injected into my right breast to make the lymph nodes easy to find.

Will I wake up tomorrow minus three lymph nodes? Or, like my neighbor Orly, minus twenty-four? That can't be known today, and I don't need to know. Today is a beautiful blue-sky day, and that's all I need to know for now.

The future, the follow-up cannot be known. It won't even be known after surgery, until pathology makes its report next week.

Meanwhile, I am starting a month-long silent retreat on Sunday, and the surgeon is taking a two-week skiing vacation in Utah. How glorious!

Sitting with the unknown.

Sitting with Life.

Going Public

FOR THE FIRST week after I received my diagnosis of breast cancer, I told only a few people. My sister—who immediately made an appointment for a mammogram, which she had let slide for the past four years. My two cousins who had had breast cancer seventeen years ago; and my other six female cousins. I had been certain that Wilfong genes were healthy genes, but now I wasn't so sure. I told my friends who had had breast cancer. I told my morning meditation group of five neighbors. I didn't tell my neighbor Connie, who holds my durable power of attorney for health care; she was on a bird-watching trip in Cuba and off the grid of cyber-communication. Nor did I tell my stepdaughter, who was on vacation with her family in St. Lucia. Interrupting her holidays just didn't seem fair.

Then on Wednesday, before my Thursday surgery, I went public—I blogged about breast cancer on TheMeditativeGardener.blogspot.com and posted it to Facebook, LinkedIn, and Twitter. I wrote about it in my Wednesday morning writing group, just after I had gone into the bathroom and applied lidocaine to numb my right nipple. The radiation department would be injecting nuclear isotopes at noon that day so that my lymph nodes would show up during surgery.

I was limiting my public exposure to about twenty-four hours before the surgery. By the time most people could respond, I would have the answers to my questions and would be better able to fend off well-meaning commiseration. Then, after my surgery, I would have only forty-eight hours of public exposure before I went into the seclusion of a month-long retreat.

I had already met a couple of women by accident at the hospital. Sheila was just walking out of the Nurse Navigator's office when I walked in. In an instant, we both knew. "Don't tell Bella that I have breast cancer," Sheila said to me, referring to a mutual friend. "I'm not quite ready to tell her myself."

The evening after I saw Imogene at the hospital, she called me and said, "I won't tell anyone that I saw you at the hospital today." She was really saying that she didn't want *me* to tell anyone that I had seen *her* at the hospital. Imogene didn't want people's sympathy. She didn't want people meeting her on the street and responding to her as if she had a big orange C on her forehead.

Some people think that problems are private. They just don't feel comfortable sharing their intimate experience. Suddenly they feel exposed. For those people who like to conform to society's norms, suddenly finding oneself outside the range of normal life and feeling like an outsider is hard. Suddenly they are a pariah among healthy friends. Will their friends shun them? Whisper about them? Talk about them behind their backs? Pity them?

People intend to commiserate, to swim together with

the afflicted person in the misery of cancer, but I wasn't feeling miserable. Coping with other people's misreadings feels awkward. Perhaps it is better not to tell people, so that you don't have to deal with their advice.

People misread us and project their own fears onto us. To the person who said, "Oh, that's terrible," I was suddenly in the position of having to comfort her. I'm sure her intention was to comfort me, but her own terror of the terribleness of cancer shifted the focus of the conversation to her.

Some friends said to me, "Oh, how awful," when I didn't feel that having cancer was so awful. Awe-full is more like it. I was awed by the smoothness and ease of the process of diagnosis and treatment.

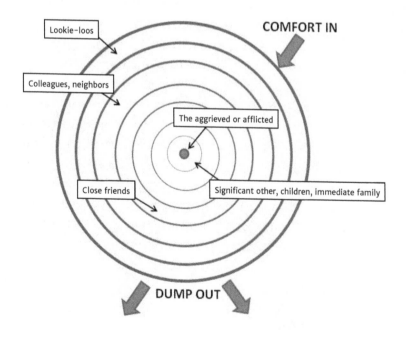

"Comfort in, vent out"[*] is a shorthand mnemonic for responding to people in distress. Think of a series of concentric circles with the stressed person being in the center. The next circle around that is close family, the next circle is close friends, et cetera. Our game plan should be to direct comfort inward from our own particular circle to the inner circles. If we need to vent, then we should direct our feelings outward to someone in our own circle (of acquaintances, for example) or further out to the circle of community or the circle of professionals.

For some, emotions can be raw. Some people are ashamed to cry, even when they are shedding tears of joy. They dash the tears from their eyes, and say, "I'm sorry. I'm sorry." I hope I never apologize for having tears of joy or my own genuine tears of grief.

I am practicing tearing up and even crying in public, because I have seen how Bill sometimes unexpectedly gets a quaver in his voice and a tear in his eye when he is sincerely expressing appreciation or showing deep feeling to or about someone. In that moment, he feels so real, so genuine, so authentic that his audience—the local Rotary Club, for example—comes to complete attention regarding his sincerity. He is not speaking ordinary, gratuitous phrases (which he and we are completely capable of); his heart is speaking. His tender heart speaks and the listener's heart vibrates in response as the other person hears and, even more importantly, *feels* the truth of the moment.

---

[*] Illustration by Eileen Tully https://littlewingedones.wordpress.com/2013/08/28/grieving-other-losses-part-2

I, too, want to speak from my vulnerable heart. I want to speak from the heart of cancer, which is neither terrible nor demonic, neither awful nor a fight. I felt it was important to go public, partly to puncture the scariness of cancer and to let people in on the inside story. We talk about our other ailments, sometimes *ad nauseam*. Why not talk about cancer?

Going public was another way for me to be honest. I value honesty very highly. I have been hurt by lies and secrets, especially in my twenties and thirties. In most movies and plays, the drama and suspense depend on the unsaid thing—the lie, the secret. I've had enough drama in my life. I don't want to have secrets, though I will keep your secret for the rest of my life, if you ask me to.

In the name of being polite, my mother allowed herself to be straitjacketed by the stigmas of the 1950s about divorce and psychotherapy, for example, neither of which she could avail herself of for another thirty years. Cancer would have been impossible for her to confront openly. She couldn't even talk about pregnancy (during the baby boom!) without using code words.* I want to demystify this bogeyman of cancer, which, in the twentieth century, was shoved in the closet as The Big C. I want to raise awareness, my own included.

Some friends call my writing TMI—too much information. They don't want to hear the gory details

---

* In 1952 (when my mother already had three children), the *I Love Lucy* sitcom could not use the word *pregnant* because the word was deemed too vulgar by CBS executives. Lucy is hilarious as she tries to tell her husband that she's pregnant (on TV! A first!) without using the word *pregnant*.

of aging and illness. I am sending a telegram to those younger than me; whether they decide to read it and heed it is their business. The young and even the middle-aged have seldom listened to the tap-tap-tap of the Heavenly Messengers lightly knocking on the door of their awareness. I'm going public with the Heavenly Messengers; I'm going public with cancer. Those who have ears will hear.

Facebook

I SIGNED UP FOR Facebook in 2009, just as people my age were catching on to it. For the first year, I used it the way anyone does, but then, with the publication of *The Meditative Gardener* in January 2010, I began to use Facebook as a marketing tool. I have to say, Facebook has failed rather spectacularly in that regard; I only receive about one order a month for my book via Facebook.

Since 2010, I've friended—added to my list of Facebook connections—every person I've met just once, maybe just for five minutes. As a result, I now have 2,000 "friends." You may scoff, but I find this Facebook friend thing to be quite amazing. I friended Cora because she ran a program for underprivileged women in Bellows Falls, a formerly thriving town twenty miles north of me. I admired her work, but I'd never actually met her. Then, in January 2014, in Oaxaca, Mexico, I was sitting at the Oaxaca Lending Library, waiting to hear an archaeology lecture, when a woman walked up to me and said, "It's The Meditative Gardener! Cheryl Wilfong!" That was Cora.

This is what Facebook friends do—recognize each other in the parking lot. "Hi, Cheryl," someone says. "We're Facebook friends." I smile and feel friendly toward this sort-of-new-to-me person. Now I have a new friend-in-the-flesh, not just a Facebook "friend."

Every day I post an entry for The Meditative Gardener blog to Facebook. For a long while, I was quite frustrated by Facebook's metrics: "23 people have seen this post." How could that be? I have a thousand followers on The Meditative Gardener's Facebook page, and only twenty-three people saw this post?

Meanwhile, once every week or so, I am stopped in a parking lot or in a store. "Oh, I saw your blog post on Facebook. It's such an inspiration. Thank you." This person is one of the twenty-three who read my post? And next week's person is one of nineteen people who "saw this post"? I had my doubts about Facebook. I began to think that by giving me such low statistics, they wanted me to buy an ad on Facebook. I began to distrust Facebook. They might not have my best interests at heart, but rather their own bottom line.

Going public with my cancer diagnosis and progress on Facebook won me a lot of support from friends near and far. Many women came up to me, in Pilates class, in the food co-op, or on the street to offer their own experience with breast cancer and say, "If there's anything I can do to help. . . ." Just knowing that these acquaintances cared was enough to warm my heart. My support network was far wider and deeper than I had suspected.

And if you ask me whether the world is friendly or hostile, I'd have to say friendly. After all, I have more than 2,000 friends. Thanks to Facebook.

Radioactive Isotopes and the Gamma Ray Camera

THE DAY BEFORE surgery, I made a quick trip into the hospital to have nuclear medicine injected into my right breast. I had already applied lidocaine around my nipple as a topical anesthetic, so I didn't feel the prick of the needle, just a slight pressure.

These particular radioactive isotopes have an affinity for lymph nodes. Lymph nodes look like translucent tapioca curds, so they are hard for the surgeon to see. But once they are radioactivated, the surgeon can hold a Geiger counter to the breast to find these little getaway cars for cancer cells.

After the injection, I sat in the waiting room for half an hour while the isotopes began cruising around my breast.

Soon enough, I was lying down under a gamma-ray camera to verify that the isotopes had been injected properly and were indeed making their journey toward the lymph nodes.

Because the word *radioactive* conjures up fallout from bombs, and pollution from nuclear power plants, the medical profession has renamed such procedures "nuclear medicine." The purpose of this radioactivity, like that of x-rays and mammograms, is to detect what can't be seen with the naked eye. In German, the word *Gift* means "poison." Sometimes we take poison, such as radiation and chemotherapy, as medicine, for the gift of a cure.

I felt happy, because this procedure meant that the surgery really would happen tomorrow. I had been lightly holding my breath, half anticipating a hiccup in the process that might, for some unpredictable reason, delay my surgery. Now there was no turning back. All systems were "go" as the radioactive isotopes were going directly to my lymph nodes.

Bill's Not Worried

AT FIRST, I thought Bill didn't really understand the seriousness of my diagnosis. Or maybe it was that he was busy with his own afflictions. He had been itching for three months with a rash, and the dermatologist was trying one thing and then another. First, Dr. Smith thought he might have folliculitis, a form of dermatitis, from the hot tub. He stopped going out to the hot tub. Or maybe he was allergic to chromium—in vitamins and leather and black dyes. So he stopped taking his vitamins.

To me, his rash looked like eczema, so I bought him three salves for eczema, and one of them brought him relief. Still, he was dotted with dime- and quarter-size red splotches all over his body, except on his face and feet. The splotches on his butt were mirror images of each other. Were those on meridians? I tried to get him to go to an acupuncturist.

Then Dr. Smith thought he might have scabies, even though I, sleeping with Bill in the same bed, had no similar symptoms. We went through three rounds of washing all our clothes and bedsheets every day, and applying permethrin, a strong insect and tick repellent cream, to our bodies at night.

Then the doctor did allergy tests on his skin, but the patches didn't stick to his hairy back. Then she thought he might be allergic to fragrances. He bought fragrance-free detergent and fragrance-free soap. Then she thought he might be allergic to cinnamon and vanilla. I changed my granola recipe. Then she thought he might have a nickel allergy. By this time, I was really ready for Bill to get a second opinion at Dartmouth-Hitchcock, but he loves his dermatologist. He canceled the appointment I'd made for him.

When we looked back, we remembered that Bill had complained of occasional bug bites in bed for a couple of years. He would wake up in the morning with "bug bites," though I had none.

Bill is a somatic guy—his emotions manifest as body ailments. So, for a while, I thought he was focusing on his own body as a roundabout way of focusing on his feelings about my cancer. Maybe he got itchy just thinking about me being sick? Was he shifting his and my focus from me to him? Did he want to be the baby of the family instead of babying me?

I really thought the penny had not dropped. But then I came up with a new theory: Bill wasn't worried, because I wasn't worried. Worry can be contagious; he wasn't "catching it" from me. Some people learn worry from their parents. Some people worry because the people around them are worrying, and they begin to wonder whether they should be worrying too.

As far as Bill was concerned, I had an illness, and the doctors would take care of it. (Better than how his dermatologist was taking care of him, I hoped!) Bill puts his faith in his doctors, and, right now, my faith is in my surgeon.

Unsolicited Advice

EVERYONE KNOWS THAT people in distress receive all sorts of unsolicited advice. I have dispensed a lot of misplaced compassion myself; now it was my turn to receive some of my own medicine. My goal was to smile—genuinely—and say "thank you" from my heart. Thank you for caring about me. Thank you for worrying about me. My other unspoken intention was to respond compassionately. *I know you are scared—scared for me and scared for yourself. But don't worry. Have no fear, because your fear does neither of us any good.*

Fair, who cleans my house, made sure I was up to date on my antioxidants. She particularly likes one you've never heard of—microhydrin—because it hydrates the body with ions. I dutifully take it, and feel that I'm getting off easy. She could recommend (as she has in the past) wearing magnets or testing the pH of my saliva every day with litmus paper. And she might have a point there, because cancer acidifies the body.

Bill read an article in the newspaper about how doctors overdiagnose and overtreat. He had so much confidence in my immune system that he wasn't sure that

I actually did have cancer. "Are you really sure you need to do this?" he asked me, just days before my surgery.

"Yes, Bill. I have confidence in this surgeon."

Some friends cared enough to stay awake half the night worrying about me because I did not get a second opinion. Others begged me not to do radiation. A couple of friends who had had breast cancer warned me not to take any of the anti-cancer drugs, because "they're so bad for you."

By offering their particular brand of fix-it advice, my friends were trying to be helpful. This is what I call "misplaced compassion." My fix-it friends were also trying to assuage their own anxiety about being sick or having cancer themselves. I've done this myself many, many times. I can now catch myself when I hear myself say, "You should . . ." or "Why don't you . . . ?"

When I hear about a friend's distress, my heart goes out to them. And my mind becomes reactive. This reactivity is another expression of my own stress and suffering. *I don't want them to suffer.* So I immediately try to fix it by offering some advice. I hear that they have a problem; I solve the problem for them. *Aren't I good? And oh-so-helpful.* Notice that my focus is on me and my darn ego again. When I'm giving advice, what I'm really doing is dealing with my own anxiety that I don't feel at all and, thus, am unaware of. Actually, I'm easing *my own* suffering, though I fail to notice that.

The Buddha says that compassion has a near enemy of pity—a mimic that looks like compassion, but is actually fake compassion, or what I am calling misplaced compassion.

True compassion wants the other person to be free from suffering. Misplaced compassion, the near enemy, wants *me* to be free from suffering, and, oh yes, the other person too. True compassion taps in to our big and wise heart that can hold the other person's suffering without commiserating with them. Counterfeit compassion commiserates.

Our friends want us to get better. They want us to be healthy, not only for our sakes, but also because being sick reminds them that their own bodies are on the downhill slide of aging, disease, and, eventually, dying. As long as we are all well, or well enough, we can keep up the illusion of beautiful, functional bodies. This illusion worked pretty well during our twenties, thirties, and forties, when we and everyone we knew were healthy, and we desperately want to hang on to it in our fifties. The illusion becomes rather tattered when we are in our sixties, and next to useless in our seventies as we recognize the moment-to-moment fragility of life.

When we become sick or diseased, we are holding up a mirror to our friends. They can really be of service to us if they have the fortitude to look, and to think to themselves: *I, too, am of the nature to get cancer. In fact, it may be that I already have it and don't know it.* This seemingly morbid thought is the birthplace of actual compassion.

True friends can sit still and listen. The simple act of paying attention can be transformative.

My neighbor Jane, a therapist, invited me over for a cup of tea. In her gentle way, she asked a few questions and listened attentively without interrupting me. She offered no advice. In her presence, I was able to touch a tiny, tender spot that had no words, just a single tear.

We want friends who can accept us just as we are, without fixing us, so that we ourselves can accept ourselves, complete with cancer, just as we are.

The enemy of compassion, the obvious enemy, is anger and hatred. If we hate cancer, if we think it is terrible or a demon, then the path to our natural compassion is blocked by the fear underlying the anger. If we are angry because we or our friends have cancer (*It's just not fair!*), then our compassion cannot flow. True compassion has an element of equanimity. Equanimity means not resisting. Equanimity means accepting things as they are.

Well, my dear, here we are.

Listen. Breathe. Pause. Don't speak into the stillness of the unknown. Allow the unknown to work on you, through you. Feel your heart. Put your hand on your heart and gaze into your friend's eyes. Pray, if praying works for you.

We all want the freedom to make our own decisions. We want autonomy, a sense of agency, over our own lives rather than advice from our friends about what we *should* do. And we want the companionship of a friend who can hold our hand and walk with us down the dark street of the unknown.

Victim?

AM I THE victim of cancer? Is cancer the persecutor? If I'm the victim, then I need a rescuer. Some friends try to rescue me from cancer with all sorts of good advice. Their unstated premise is "I can help you."

"Wanting to help" is the top of a slippery slope because it often springs from the impulse to save the other person so that they will need us. Trying to save someone looks and feels so much like compassion, yet it's just a little off-key. It means that I, the healthy one, am standing outside trying to help you, the sick one, and maybe looking down on you, poor thing.

I would add acting like a do-gooder or trying to be a rescuer to the list of forms of faux compassion. The do-gooder or the rescuer is left with the self-satisfied feeling of yes-I-know-how-to-help-you-if-you-would-just-do-what-I-tell-you-to-do.

Let's say I feel fear, worry, or grief when my friend is ill or dying or has cancer. To make an end run and reduce my own anxiety (which I'm not even aware of feeling), I go straight into problem solving, straight into fix-it mode. I love being Ms. Fix-It. But fixing it has a shadow side—it puts me in the one-up position, and it puts the sick person, the distressed person, in the one-down position. In transactional analysis language, I act like the parent, thereby reducing the distressed person to a child role. While this "helping" is pretty comfortable for my own ego, the recipient is not really "helped."

"You should . . ." obscures my open heart. "You should . . ." or "you shouldn't . . ." is a you-statement. Let me back up and begin again with an I-statement: "I feel. . . ." Let's have a heart-to-heart instead of a head-to-head. Chances are that what "I feel" is so uncomfortable that I just want to get away from it.

As a once-upon-a-time therapist, I try to avoid being either the victim or, more likely, the rescuer. A victim is a sorry sight, someone who should be pitied. A victim is a powerless person. A victim is not responsible. Something terrible happened to her. Then along come well-meaning friends who want to be the Lone Ranger, ride to the rescue, and recommend their silver-bullet remedies. Ever so subtly, this shifts the focus to the rescuer. A rescuer *needs* to have a victim in order for the rescuer to be the good guy.

It's hard to watch people suffer, and harder still to watch our friends and loved ones shoot themselves in the foot with unwise actions. These situations call for our compassion. We are not their savior. Each person is responsible for the consequences of their actions, despite our best wishes for them.

People used to say "cancer victim," back when the cure rate was low. But now, survivors far outnumber cancer victims, almost two to one. Now, the cancer lingo has shifted to "survivor." As a survivor, I need your compassion and support so that I can thrive. I don't need to be "saved" from cancer.

Let go of the idea of victim of cancer. Let go of the idea of victory over cancer. I want to be a thriving survivor, surfing this windy river of life.

Company and Parting Company

O N T H E M O R N I N G of my surgery, I had to be at the hospital at 7:30, though my surgery wasn't scheduled until 11:00. The future doesn't exist, except as an idea, but one way the concept of the future is very useful is that we meet at an agreed-upon time and place. Today, I would meet the surgeon at the hospital.

Bill, a late riser, got up at 6:30 to go with me. I was ready, really ready to go as I drove into the overcast, eleven-degree morning, while he relaxed in the reclined passenger's seat for the twenty-minute ride. That rascal breast cancer and I were just about to part company. I was looking forward to being lighter by one ounce of breast tissue.

Bill and I walked to the outpatient care unit, where I disrobed, put on a johnny, and met my very own nurse, Victoria, dressed in blue scrubs, who braceleted me in orange plastic with my name and birth date. Dr. Rosen dropped by in his blue scrubs to say hello and to meet Bill.

At 8:30, I was ferried over to the radiology depart-ment in a wheelchair. There were Dr. Watson, the friendly radiologist who had walked me to the surgeon's office four weeks earlier, and Nurse Navigator Kelly, covered with a pretty lavender-and-pink-print lead apron. She offered her hand and chatted to keep me distracted as the radiologist, with the aid of the mammography machine, was threading a wire into my breast to guide the surgeon to X-marks-the-spot. The X was the abnormality near a tiny titanium spiral that the surgeon had inserted into my breast during the biopsy, two and a half weeks earlier. Kelly was doing her best to distract me from the little sensations of pressure, but I was fascinated by the monitor attached to the mammogram machine. How could Dr. Watson "see" in 3-D when the screen was only 2-D?

Dr. Watson then injected my nipple with a blue dye that would bind with and color the nuclear isotopes he'd injected the day before, which were now, we hoped, in my lymph nodes, turning them from translucent to blue, which would make them much easier for the surgeon to see

Then I was wheeled back to "my" room in the outpatient care unit to await my turn in the operating room. Here I was, on the hospital's "conveyor belt" of a schedule. I had no control over my forward momentum; my body was taken here and there, put here and there, and subjected to various procedures. The question then became: How does the mind cope with this lack of control, this not-knowing, this conveyor belt?

Bill's method is to chat with everyone he sees; he is expert at making small talk and loosening people up with a laugh. He likes people, and he especially likes good-looking women under the age of fifty. Although I would rather "cocoon" when I'm on the conveyor belt of the airport or the hospital, and although I'm not a natural at making momentary friends, I have learned from Bill to at least try being conversational with strangers and acting at ease. Once upon a time, I was a consultant; I know I can land on my feet in a brand-new situation. I decided to enjoy myself here in the hospital to the best of my ability.

Bill had a dermatology appointment at ten, and the idea of sitting alone in a sterile and probably cool hospital room, waiting alone, seemed rather dismal, so I had called two Dharma friends. Lani, who lives near the hospital, is a meditation-in-action gal. Her intention is to bring joy to everyone around her. I asked if she could come over and visit me for an hour before surgery, and she was happy to do so. I also called Mary, a meditation friend, whom I call our small meditation center's compassionate-care-committee-of-one. True to form, Mary said she was bringing Evelyn, our meditation center's former volunteer administrator, to the hospital that morning at 9:30 for chemo. She would be waiting for Evelyn for an hour.

Perfect, I thought. "Can you come visit me while you're waiting for Evelyn?" I asked.

Mary said she'd be happy to come visit me.

I felt exhilarated that plans were proceeding without a hitch. Having some company in my hospital room would make the morning more jolly, and the time would pass more quickly.

Lani arrived first, and Bill gave her the comfortable chair across from me. Mary arrived a few minutes later, and Bill left for his appointment.

Effervescent Lani is so entertaining that the energy in a room starts to bubble when she walks in. She talked about her upcoming month-long trip to Panama to do some birding. Lani has been to all seven continents and loves to travel alone. She meets the most amazing people, learns one song from every country she visits, and sometimes just walks into local people's kitchens and makes herself at home. She has made herself at home in my home, and, as a result, I feel at home with her, no matter where in the world we are.

I brought Lani and Mary up to date on the various procedures I had been through. Mary spoke of her ongoing search to buy a house. We were having such a good time that I forgot to fret when my scheduled surgery time of 11:00 came and went.

Bill returned, and Mary went to pick up Evelyn. Lani dashed off to do an errand. At 11:30 I met the anesthesiologist, Dr. Todd, who was half my age. I didn't really notice that, as we talked, he was injecting something into the IV. And then, suddenly, I was asleep.

I Woke Up Wearing a Bra

WHEN I WOKE up, three hours later, I was wearing a bra. Wow! How did that happen? I tried to imagine nurses putting a bra on me as I slept, sort of rag-doll fashion. Then I dozed off for a few minutes, but Victoria, my outpatient-care nurse, woke me up to tell me the good news: my sentinel lymph node, the node nearest the tumor, was clear of cancer. Dr. Rosen had taken two additional lymph nodes, and they too were clear. She handed me a sheet of paper with the times of the pathology report on the lymph nodes—1:25, 1:28, and 1:32. Three clear lymph nodes!

I was ready to skip to the front door of the hospital, but they had to put me in a wheelchair to discharge me.

I was fascinated with the bra, since I hadn't worn one in decades. First of all, I was feeling a lot more buxom than 34B. Where did that cleavage come from? I soon deduced that the bra was holding my traumatized, swollen breast together. I tried to sleep without the bra—for about two minutes. Then I put it back on, and kept it on, day and night, for a week. I did take it off in order to shower at night, but then put it right back on, under my nightgown.

The soft, stretchy, cotton-and-nylon surgical bra was also holding my steri-strip in place—a narrow, nearly transparent, two-inch-long tape, sort of a band-aid that covered the incision on the right side of my right breast. A shorter steri-strip covered the lymph node incision in my underarm.

I was thrilled that my new bra velcroed together in the front. The last bra I wore, all those years earlier, had underwires and three hooks-and-eyes in the middle of my back, which were impossible to reach even in the days when I had shoulder flexibility.

Over the next few days, the Velcro began to irritate my cleavage, so I loosened the Velcro at the top and velcroed the scratchy top edges back onto the bra fabric. If the bra hadn't been covered by my woolen undershirt, a merino wool shirt, and a fleece sweater, I would have looked rather risqué.

After wearing that bra day and night for a week, then during the day for another few days, I tucked it into the back of my underwear drawer. I haven't looked at it since.

Brava for that bra.

Surrendering to Life #2

WHEN I SAY I am surrendering to Life, I am not talking about a belief. I am not believing in Fate and telling others that "It must have been meant to be like that." I am not taking a spiritual bypass and pretending that things are hunky-dory.

No. I am talking about watching the in-breath of Life and its out-breath, attending to the hills and valleys of Life with equipoise, neither wanting the better nor not wanting the worse.

Life unfolds, moment by moment. I have no decisions to make. Not really. When the time comes, the decisions make themselves without me.

You could say I am on the hospital's conveyor belt. It rolls along like this, and I find myself at the second mammogram. Then I am walking beside the radiologist to the surgeon's office. Then he is saying, "She wants an appointment with Dr. Rosen." I do? The decision has been made for me. The surgeon puts me on his calendar. And then I wake up from anesthesia, and they tell me three lymph nodes are clear. The process rolls on, and I am processed by the system, which, I thank my lucky stars, is working wonderfully well.

Fortunately, I've already made the decision to do a month-long retreat in March at home, instead of flying to Arizona to sit with an awakened teacher or flying to California to a Byron Katie retreat. I would have to cancel those plane reservations because I'm not supposed to fly for two weeks after surgery. I'm so happy I didn't make the reservations in the first place.

Someone calls this lucky decision the result of listening to my guardians and guides. Perhaps. My retreat is bookended by surgery at the end of February and an appointment with the oncologist in early April. Just luck. Very, very good luck.

Or Life. Just flowing with Life and watching Life breathe me into and out of existence.

Even If I Did Everything Right

AFTER THE GOOD news of my surgery, when I was safe and sound at home, that's when an incarnation of fear arose. I could do everything right—make the right treatment decisions, eat the right foods, get the right exercise—and still cancer could grab my breast and say, "Hey, lady, you're coming with me."

I don't know. I don't know. Not knowing.

I love knowing. I hate not knowing. Yet here I am—square in the middle of not knowing.

Sure, I can rely on statistics and probability, but wanting to know the unknowable, wanting to know but not knowing, lands me face to face with the fact of uncertainty and the equally uncomfortable *feeling* of uncertainty, as well as the pushy feeling of wanting, wanting. Wanting to know. Wanting life. Not wanting cancer.

The Buddha called this wanting "craving." It's the Second Noble Truth, which he simply called *tanha* or "thirst." I think of the thirst of the alcoholic, which is craving in stark relief. An unquenchable thirst. My wanting, wanting to know, is unquenchable, because what is not known cannot be known.

I want to know what's right. I want to know the future as if that would enable me to make the best decision right now. What a mind twister!

The Buddha called the Third Noble Truth *cessation*. I am ceasing hostilities with cancer. I cease wanting life to go *my* way. Sometimes, I cease the fire of wanting, wanting, and I become interested in the mystery of not-knowing. At other times, I recognize the internal stress of wanting, wanting, wanting to know, and I label that openness "mindfulness of the present moment."

In doing everything as "right" as I can, I am setting up the conditions for my karma as best I can. This is what we do when we make lifestyle changes. We already believe, more or less, in the cause and effect that is karma. By changing our diet and our exercise patterns, we are attempting to set up a different outcome for our bodies We already have a pretty good idea where the habits of smoking and drinking, of junk food and soda pop, are going to lead.

Typically, we think of karma as the results of our actions, but the word *karma* means action, intentional action, deliberate action. After one has repeated an action a few times, the track is laid, the habit is formed, the neural pathway is greased. Our automatic action (karma) is now a habit (also karma). The karma, the action, the habit of smoking is probably, but not certainly, going to lead to an unhealthy body as a consequence of our choices. Since our future is "born" from our current action, it's best for us, and for the people around us, if we choose our words wisely and act skillfully right now, in the present moment.

We all know people who live a clean life and still get cancer. Karma is not tit-for-tat. The Buddha said that trying to figure out the complexities of karma will drive you crazy. Blaming people for their cancer ("It must be your karma") is extremely uncompassionate.

In addition to karma, our bodies are subject to the laws of the natural world—we might call this genetics, we might call it the nature of each particular body. The laws of the natural world may prevail over an individual's karma. I really have no idea how nature and nurture are going to play out in my body. I do the best I can, and that's the best I can do. I might do everything right, and still, cancer might win my body.

The body ages, becomes sick, and eventually dies of something or other. My mind will be with me until the very end of my decrepit body, and depending on your beliefs, perhaps beyond. How about changing the "lifestyle" of my mind? What if I spent at least as much time working on my habits of mind as I do working out my body?

Knowing that cancer may prevail over my body at any time, I recommit to my spiritual development. Now is the time to build kindness, compassion, love, gratitude, contentment, and calm. Then, whatever happens, life or death, my mind is prepared, not with strategies and not with a plan of action, but with an acceptance of life as it is unfolding in the present moment.

ON RETREAT:
Healing from Surgery

Self-Retreat at Home

Two days after my lumpectomy, I started my previously scheduled five-week retreat.

Thirteen years ago, I made a commitment to myself to go on a month-long retreat every year to support my spiritual practice and deepen my insight into the Dharma. I had negotiated an understanding with Bill that he could indeed survive for a month without me. I viewed these retreats partly as a death-practice. One of these days, Bill will be living alone without me, or I will be living alone without him. This "separate vacation" (though I would hardly call a retreat a "vacation") is a way of practicing for this eventuality.

This year, instead of going far away, I had decided to do my first-ever at-home self-retreat.

Knowing that the day would come when Bill would be too old for me to go away for my month-long retreats, I had a guest suite—"The Sweet"—built on the back side of our new two-car garage. Bedroom, sitting room, galley kitchen, and a completely accessible bathroom mean that this suite could be our old-age bedroom when that day comes. I imagine being able to push Bill in a wheelchair from the garage into The Sweet and straight into the shower—no thresholds—where I can hose him off while he hangs onto grab bars. In the meantime, it's our guest suite and a great place to have committee meetings or workshops. And it's listed on Airbnb as "The Sweet for Sweethearts," so we have paying guests a couple of times a month. For three weeks during the month of March, I would be retreating to The Sweet for several hours of meditation each day; then I was going to a retreat center for another two weeks.

Going to a retreat center locks you into their schedule, which is very helpful. Doing a self-retreat has the advantage of a freer schedule and the disadvantage of perhaps being a little too free.

One of the benefits of any retreat is that I can actually sleep for eight hours at a time. All that meditating clears the clutter out of the corners of my mind, so I don't wake up at zero-dark-thirty turning something over and over in my mind. On this self-retreat, I simply woke up at about 5:30, rolled out of bed, and went downstairs to stoke the fire in the woodstove. I did my first meditation on the sofa in our living room, as I usually do when I'm at home. By this time, dawn would be breaking, so I walked thirty feet on the icy sidewalk over to The Sweet Retreat to turn up the heat, have a cup of tea, and do my next forty-five-minute sit.

I usually meditate with my neighbors at eight o'clock. While on retreat, I was not venturing out into the world, not even walking to my neighbor's house. However, one of my neighbors, Connie, got into the habit of coming to The Sweet at eight for meditation. Connie and I began meditating together once a week when we were thirty. Two years later, when she had her first child, our practice fell away, but when she turned fifty, we started sitting together again every morning. Nineteen years later, our meditation group included four other neighbors as well. Those other four were meditating every weekday morning at Lynn's house.

On this retreat, Connie and I would practice one of the new chants I was trying to learn. We limited our conversation. "I'm not going to ask you about your bird-watching trip to Cuba," I told her. "That will have to wait until next month." While she was in the tropics, she had missed my diagnosis and surgery, so she was catching up on me—but the details of that, too, would have to wait.

After Connie left, I would eat a simple breakfast of granola. Then I would do a household chore.

Later, I joked that Bill-the-extrovert did not take a vow of silence. What really happened was that I did not take a vow of silence with Bill. I had silenced my phone, silenced my e-mail with the automatic response that "I will return from retreat in early April." I silenced my reading, and I silenced my writing. I silenced my driving—I was not going grocery shopping or anywhere. But I did not silence Bill-the-relational-guy. For this he was extremely grateful.

At about 9:30 A.M., I would return to my retreat for a

couple of sitting periods before lunch. That left me about half an hour for yoga stretches and half an hour to chop ice off the sidewalk or shovel snow or, my favorite chore, to play in my solarium, taking cuttings from house plants or potting them up.

Lunch at The Sweet Retreat was also simple—either soup that a neighbor had brought over, post-surgery, or one of those Indian meals in a foil packet that you drop into boiling water for a couple of minutes.

After a nap, I sat for a couple of periods in the afternoon, interspersed with more chores and probably more talking with Bill, if he was home. On some chilly afternoons, I would strap studded-snow-tires-for-your-feet onto my boots and walk back and forth in the driveway, doing walking meditation for twenty minutes.

I refrained from eating dinner, though I might have a rice cake or a cracker with hummus. Limiting food during a retreat helps keep my mind sharp, because food usually translates into sleepiness later. Bill was on his own in the kitchen, thawing out leftovers from the freezer.

Evenings were the most difficult. My mind was tired. I could manage a half-hour sit, and I often listened to guided meditations. I tried listening to Dharma talks by various teachers, but I was uninspired. So I tried to learn a new chant as a way to keep myself occupied and out of the house.

At 9:30 P.M. I would return to the house and go to bed.

Bill had requested that I sleep with him, but I was

in bed before him, and I awoke long before he did, so there wasn't much opportunity for pillow talk. Bill does like to report to me on his day at about 10:00 P.M., just as my eyes are at half-mast. I had warned him, and he knew from previous experience, that I didn't want him to tell me any news or the plots of any TV programs he was watching.

Every four days, I would have a forty-five-minute phone call with Doreen, a Dharma friend and the guiding teacher at Valley Insight Meditation Society, an hour north in Lebanon, New Hampshire, to talk about my practice.

I am still always amazed at how much the mind calms down when I pare my life down to the basics. The avalanche of information that normally comes into my eyes and ears every day stimulates my body and my mind more than I am aware of. When I renounce the superfluous, almost all the supports for my ego—phone, e-mail, reading, writing—are put on hold. Even though I was only thirty feet away from the playground of my computer, I could have been out in the middle of nowhere. Since I live in the backwoods at the end of a dirt road, some people think I already live in the boondocks.

Pause. This is the first step to mindfulness. Pause the reactive mind. Breathe. Notice that you are breathing.

For one month, I was pausing in the middle of my life, pausing in mid-stride, pausing the inflow of information, pausing the outflow of me, me, me. Treating myself to a retreat.

My First Retreat

I WENT ON MY first ten-day retreat as my thirtieth birthday present to myself. The previous summer, a passing acquaintance had said to me, "Hey, there's this new retreat center in Barre, Massachusetts—just an hour from here. You should go."

The reason I considered it was that I thought that watching my breath would be very handy the next time I had an asthma attack.

In the spring of that year, 1977, I had had an asthma attack severe enough to put me into the hospital for four days. It scared my parents enough that they flew out to be with me. I had had debilitating asthma as a child, but this was only my third attack as an adult, and the first time that asthma had ever landed me in the hospital.

So, after Christmas 1977, I drove down to the Insight Meditation Society. The teachers were all about my age—Joseph Goldstein, Jack Kornfield, Sharon Salzberg, and Jacqueline Schwarz. Joseph and Jack gave the Dharma talks on alternate nights. Joseph talked about the Dharma, but what I remember are Jack's talks, which were based on the Carlos Castañeda book *Journey to Ixtlan*—a book I had read seven times.

The key teachings of Don Juan, a Yaqui sorcerer, to his apprentice, Carlos, were: follow a path with heart; assume responsibility for your actions; act like a warrior; always remember that death is your adviser, your eternal companion, at arm's length, to your left.

It was as a result of taking responsibility for my actions that I had started meditating five years earlier, after I had fallen into a black pit of depression, accompanied, at times, by severe anxiety. Over the course of several months, I meditated my way out of the depression. What kept me meditating for twenty minutes every morning was the relief it gave me from anxiety—sometimes just five minutes of relief, but on some days, five hours. *Ahhh.*

I was really preferring this insight meditation to my previous practice of psychosynthesis meditation. The latter uses a lot of beautiful imagery, visualizations, and affirmations, but I kept feeling I was slapping a veneer of love and peace over my punky heartwood of anger and self-loathing. With psychosynthesis, I felt that I was somehow lying, because, at heart, I was unlovable and, sometimes, even unlikable. Although psychosynthesis calls itself a psychology of hope, deep down I felt I was a hopeless case. The simple nonjudgmental awareness of insight meditation, on the other hand, gave rise to a very tiny joy, a true joy, uncreated by me, simply happening all by itself. I also considered myself a naturally insightful person; even the name "insight meditation" appealed to me. In fact, during this ten-day retreat, I had the insight that mindfulness would be a very good skill to have with me on my deathbed. To that end, I should practice mindfulness daily.

I had found my path with heart—insight meditation.

P.S. I never had another asthma attack.

Clear Margins

THREE DAYS INTO my retreat at home, I got into my car and drove to the hospital for an appointment with Nurse Navigator Kelly.

She clicked into my electronic records, and reported, "Clear margins."

Whew!

"Three millimeters," she said. "That means it was three millimeters from the edge to the cancerous tissue. Around here, three millimeters is as good as a country mile."

I smiled.

"LCIS," she said.

I grinned. Lobular Carcinoma In Situ (LCIS). Most breast cancers are in the ducts of the breast, but mine had been in a lobe. Just one lobe. "In situ" means that it had not broken through the wall of the lobe to glom onto other nearby tissue. It was contained within itself.

I fairly danced out of Kelly's office, down the stairs, and out into the snowy month of March.

Now I could settle into my retreat. No more phone calls. No more e-mails. No more worries.

I cleared out the margins of my life, simplifying it down to the basics—sitting, walking, eating, sleeping. Simply living and happy to be simply alive.

Cancer-Free

CANCER HAD BEEN growing undetected in my body for between five and nine years. It was slowly doubling in size every hundred or so days, until, finally, it was big enough to be seen on a mammogram.

I look at the photo on my driver's license, taken seven years ago. That woman, that Cheryl, thought, "Cancer doesn't run in my family." "I have a strong immune system." "I don't have any chronic disease, even if other people my age do." That woman was proud of her health. That woman thought her health, her body was under her control. That woman was deluded.

Despite those thoughts, despite those beliefs, cancer cells were already coagulating in her right breast, her Amazon breast. She thought she was an Amazon, a strong woman. Other people got sick, other people had diseases, but not her.

Many undetectable cancers are making homes for themselves in our bodies right now. We can live peacefully with some of them for decades. They behave, and we think we are home free—free from cancer.

No longer am I deluded enough to think that *free* means "free." *Free* only means undetectable; it does not mean I am exempt from future cancer. "Free" might be a permanent state, but, then again, it might be temporary.

One of my meditation teachers, Ayya Khema, had breast cancer for fourteen years. She didn't have it treated, but used it as a spur to her practice. Time is limited. One possibility is to simply live with cancer for years and years. Choose quality of life over quantity of life.

For now, I can choose both quality and (I hope) quantity. Even though the cancer has been removed with clear margins and my first three lymph nodes are free from malignancy, I'm not so short-sighted as to think that I am forever cancer-free. In fact, technically speaking, I may not be literally cancer-free at all right now. I am as "cancer-free" as the next person.

This whiff of aging and disease, the specter of eventual death, gets my attention. It's time to put first things first, and let go of the unimportant. It's time to free myself from *shoulds* and *coulds* and live in line with what's most important to me. It's time to become more truly, authentically me. There's no better time. Because, one of these days, there will be no more time. Now is the time to use my time to serve my purpose in life, to focus on my quality of life, and let the quantity of my life play its mysterious self out.

A Year to Live

A MONTH AFTER MY father died, in November 1997, I heard about a new book, *A Year to Live: How to Live This Year as if It Were Your Last* by Steven Levine. I got together a group of interested people, mostly fellow hospice volunteers, who wanted to take on the practice of living as if we had only one more year to live.

One of the women, Gladys, in her mid-sixties, had had breast cancer ten years previously. After her surgery, she had been very keenly aware of life and death and what's important, but that on-the-edginess had faded back to ordinary life. She wanted to take on this year-to-live practice as a way of renewing her attention to the facts of life and death.

I was doing it as part of my grieving process for my dad. Bob, a former minister, was interested in all things hospice. Susan, a visiting nurse, had her finger on the pulse of those in our community who were dying.

Every month we reported to each other on our assignments. Eventually, I wrote my obituary and gave it to the funeral home. They gave me laminated cards to carry in my purse and car: *In case of death, call Atamaniuk Funeral Home*. For the sake of not having regrets, I made a list of friends and family I loved and made plans to visit them, even though they lived far away. I finished unfinished business. I reviewed what was really important to me. I made my bucket list, although the term "bucket list" wouldn't enter our vocabulary for another ten years. I reviewed my will. I finally did my advance directives. Oh, did that feel good!

I "died" on the day of the winter solstice of the next year, but our group continued to meet for another two years.

One of the things that didn't quite make it into my year-to-live was going to India, so I traveled there two weeks later January. I had friends living in New Delhi who put me on the train to Bodh Gaya, where the Buddha was enlightened. I did a ten-day retreat there, then spent a week in Varanasi, a holy city for Hindus. Every day I went to the ghat along the Ganges where, in plain view, a dozen funeral pyres were burning bodies of the dead. I walked through the nearby doorless building with no glass in the windows, where very sick people lay on the floor waiting to die in this holy, smoke-filled place. I was trying to walk to the brink of death and peer over the edge.

When I returned to Ken and Jane's home in New Delhi, I wrote. And I wrote. That was the beginning of my annual booklets, each one containing a section on death. For it is only by facing death, taking death as our adviser for everything we do, that we can truly live, whether we have one day or 10,000 remaining.

The Fear-Dispelling Buddha

FOR MY FIRST two weeks in The Sweet Retreat, I set up an altar on a table. The first thing I placed on the table was a fear-dispelling Buddha—a standing Buddha holding his right hand up, palm outward, as if to say "Stop." Stop the mind, and thereby stop the fear. His left hand is down by his side, palm open, as if to say "Drop it. Just drop it. Let go. Let be."

I met the fear-dispelling Buddha while I was on my ten-day retreat in India, in early 1999. I had arrived at the retreat center, the Thai temple in Bodh Gaya, to discover that I was allergic to the entire sleeping arrangements. Straw mats. *Ah-choo.* Inch-thick kapok mattresses, which had been stored in a closet for the past year and smelled like mildew. *Ah-choo.* Mosquito nets stored in the same closet. *Ah-choo.*

I certainly didn't want to sleep in an enclosed room with all that moldy smell, so I opted to sleep on the open-air verandah, along with twenty other women. We were packed in like sardines. My sleeping nose was inches away from my neighbors' straw mats and mildewed mattresses. *Ah-choo.* I didn't want to sit in the meditation hall, because the meditation cushions had been stored in the same mattress and mosquito-net closet during last year's monsoon season. *Ah-choo!*

I left the temple and bought a new mattress, a new cushion, and a tarp to cover my neighbors' straw mats. I sent my straw mat back to the closet.

In my youth, sneezing was the precursor of wheezing and the launching pad for a weeklong suffocating asthma attack. Although I had my preventative meds with me in India, and although I went to the nurse-on-call at the retreat every morning during her office hours, I still felt terrified. My neighbor, Connie, who traveled to Southeast Asia for her work once or twice a year, had told me more than one story about American co-workers in her NGO dying of an asthma attack in Nepal or some other country. One day, I spent two forty-five-minute meditation periods outdoors sobbing with fear about my ability to breathe.

The next time I was in the meditation hall listening to a Dharma talk, I noticed a golden Buddha statue on a shelf above the teacher. From my back-row seat, near the drafty back door (fresh air!), the shiny statue looked like an Oscar. But I was pretty sure that the Buddha's first name wasn't Oscar. Eventually, the teacher mentioned that the standing Buddha was the fear-dispelling Buddha. He's been my special buddy ever since.

Although sitting Buddhas, with their hands in all sorts of positions (mudras) are quite common, it took me a week of shopping in India to find a standing, fear-dispelling Buddha. When I finally saw just such a Buddha, hand-carved, I bought it directly from the wood-carver himself.

This Buddha has gone on several retreats with me. At home, he overlooks my bed. Right after surgery, he seemed like just the right Buddha-buddy to have with me on this retreat.

La Calavera Catrina

NEXT TO THE fear-dispelling Buddha stood La Catrina—a little clay statue I had bought the previous year in Oaxaca. Catrina is dressed in a long purple evening gown. She wears a broad-brimmed purple hat with a white ostrich feather, and she carries a golden purse. All statues and mannequins of La Catrina are beautiful and ghastly. La Calavera Catrina (the dapper skeleton) is a woman in a low-cut evening dress with bulging breasts that are cut away to show a cadaver's rib cage underneath. Sometimes her skeleton arms with their long gloves are holding a cigarette or a drink, and she is often grinning or laughing, as if the joke is on us.

La Catrina symbolizes Mexico's *Dia de Muertos*, a three-day celebration when people take picnics to the graves of their loved ones and spend the day in the cemetery at a family reunion with the spirits of their dearly departed. Meanwhile, many *norteamericanos* haven't been to visit the graves of their own parents since the day of the funeral, years ago. Memorial Day is a U.S. holiday, no longer called Decoration Day, no longer meaning a day to go and decorate the family graves and remember the members of our family. Now Memorial Day just means a three-day weekend that marks the beginning of summer.

La Catrina is an excellent model of Mexico's Day of the Dead on November 1 (All Saints Day) and November 2 (All Souls Day), but she is also a perfect object for Buddhist meditation, because she epitomizes the heavenly messenger of death. Although I was repulsed by La Catrina and her Mexican skeleton cousins when I first met them in my twenties, I have recently become rather fond of skeletons depicted as dancing, drinking, or talking on mobile phones.

In La Catrina, skin, flesh, and bones are all visible. I look like that, too. I just don't see it, nor do I particularly want to see how my body breaks down into constituent parts. During this retreat, I was contemplating these very parts of the body that are so visible in La Catrina: skin—not beautiful (at least not when you look at it really closely); flesh and muscle—not beautiful; bones—not beautiful.

I was also doing a Four Elements meditation. Bones, being hard, represent the earth element. Flesh, carrying liquids of blood and lymph, represents the water element. Skin is sensitive to heat and cold and thus represents the fire element. Breath represents the air element.

All these basic so-called elements—earth, water, fire, and air—are on loan from the world around me. I say "my body," which leads me to believe that my body belongs to me. But one day, it will be payback time—time to pay back the loan and return the earth-water-fire-air of "my" body to Mother Nature. It will be time for my body or cremains to go to La Catrina's playground—the cemetery.

I undertake these contemplations on parts of the body and on the "elements" as ways to deconstruct the self and thereby undermine the ego. The mind likes its deluded belief that my body is mine. But another part of my mind really does want to know the truth.

La Catrina was originally a parody of the indigenous people who imitated European style and denied their own cultural heritage. We, too, dress our bodies in new clothes, dye our hair, and do all sorts of things to our faces as we try to distract our minds from the obvious—our bodies are aging. We try to deny the nature of our own growing-old bodies by clothing them in new and younger fashions, dying our hair, or applying "anti-aging" creams (as if anti-aging was possible).

In the end, we will all turn into a La Catrina, no matter how substantial a wardrobe we have. Death is a neutralizing force—rich and poor, we are all equal in the end. Each person carries her carcass around with her—skin, flesh, bones—composed of the four elements, which will crumble when there's no longer enough life force to bind earth, water, fire, and air together.

I kept looking at La Catrina, her strapless purple gown slipping down her ribcage as she desperately tries to hold it up and hold on to the beautiful illusion of body, my body.

Our youth-oriented culture skitters away from these reminders of death, preferring to focus on beautiful bodies, which are actually bags of skin holding together not-so-beautiful flesh and bones. La Catrina shows me this delusion of the beautiful body in stark detail. There she stood on my altar, grinning at me every time I opened my eyes after meditation.

My Altar

NEXT TO THE fear-dispelling Buddha and La Catrina, I added a mouse skeleton and a dead bird to my altar on a little table. I found the skeleton, complete with tiny toe bones, several years ago, at the bottom of a large box of camping equipment. That box was a warm, cozy home—with no exit. I, too, live in a home—my body—that has no exit, except death.

The dead bird is a vireo that I found on the terrace last summer, his beak open, his yellow and dark brown tail feathers fanned out. Beautiful.

The flowers on my altar, or in any vase, are showing us impermanence. Here today, gone tomorrow. The flowers as well as ourselves.

As an afterthought, I brought over one of my favorite statues, Nong Toranee, often found in Lao temples, and sometimes in Thai temples as well. In murals in Laos, you see the Buddha sitting in his typical enlightenment position—legs crossed in full lotus under a bodhi tree, with his right hand reaching down to touch the earth. On the night of his enlightenment, Mara, the King of Death, came to tempt the Buddha with visions of power, money, and women. The soon-to-be Buddha reached down to touch the earth, a sort of as-the-earth-is-my-witness gesture. And with that, the armies and the temptations of Mara were drowned.

In Laos, this story fits very neatly on top of the ancient animist religion. Murals in Laotian temples show the Buddha sitting on a little hillock, under the bodhi tree. Inside the little hill stands Nong Toranee, an earth spirit whom we might call Mother Nature. Nong Toranee is wringing the water out of her long, long, black hair and literally drowning the armies of Mara, the tempter.

Oh, it's so good to see a woman in the story. I was thrilled when I finally found a little silver statue of Nong Toranee in Luang Prabang when I was there a few years ago.

During my self-retreat, I focused on memorizing one chant I particularly like. One section says:

> *Through the goodness that arises from my*
> *practice . . .*
> *May the highest gods and evil forces,*
> *Celestial beings, guardian spirits of the earth, and*
> *the Lord of Death,*
> *May those who are friendly, indifferent, or hostile,*
> *May all beings receive the blessings of my life.*

I could look at my altar as I sang this chant and see a guardian spirit of the earth—Nong Toranee. And I could see the Lord (Lady, actually) of Death—La Catrina.

I could wish, every day, that all those who are friendly

to me receive the blessings of my life. May those who are indifferent to me or act indifferently because they don't know what to say to me about cancer receive the blessings of my life. May even those who are hostile to me because I rub them the wrong way and those who don't like me receive the blessings of my life. I wish, truly wish that these friends, acquaintances, and relatives—all of them—receive the blessings of my life.

A Force of Nature

I CALL CANCER A force of nature. It sweeps people away in the midst of their lives. Actually, it's more accurate to say that cancer sweeps friends away in the midst of *my* life, and what turns out to be the end of their lives.

Mark is three months older than I and has been given five months to live. My mind has a hard time comprehending this, because all during elementary school, high school, college, graduate studies, and my twenties, I assumed that my cohort and I were on the same track. Age and the grade you were in were so important for so many years, even decades, that I truly did not see that each person has her own life span.

We all had the same twelve-years-of-school life span. Then there was the four-years-of-college life span. You can see how the assumption might creep in that we'd all have the same overall chronological life span. Yet we do not. We come in together, but we do not leave together.

Cancer takes people any old (or young) time. Marilyn Fatzinger, whom I was often at odds with during my twelve years of school, died when she was thirty. Her neighbor, Barney Barton, the tallest boy in our class at six-foot-nine, died at age sixty, of prostate cancer.

Mark is spending his last summer kayaking on our local rivers and ponds. Margaret, age seventy, has cancer metastases all over her body, one of them on her pancreas. She is forty pounds lighter than she was last summer and trying to gain her strength back.

Loved ones are swept away by cancer, whether or not I am ready.

Now that I know that my own body can be a host for cancer, I take it very seriously. But I do not struggle and I do not fight. Nor do I call it "enemy." What's the use of struggling against a hurricane, fighting a blizzard, or calling a drought "enemy"?

Cancer is a force of Nature, forcing me to accept the nature of life, just as it is.

The Five Daily Reflections

For six of my month-long retreats, I have watched Ayya Khema on videotape. This Jewish German woman, who survived the Holocaust while she was in a Japanese prisoner-of-war camp in Shanghai, and who became the first Theravadin female monk in a thousand years, was quite firm about the importance of the five daily reflections. I dutifully practiced them every day for five years, and they continue to come to mind quite often:

> *I am of the nature to grow old.*
> *I am of the nature to become ill.*
> *I am of the nature to die.*
> *Everything I cherish will change and vanish.*
> *Karma is the only thing I own.*

Ayya Khema's life is quite an inspiration. Her father was one of seven brokers on the Berlin Stock Exchange, but her parents emigrated to Shanghai in late 1938. After Kristallnacht in November 1938, her parents made arrangements for her to go to England on the Kindertransport, and in April 1939, she was put on a ship bound for Dover. At age fifteen, but so short that she looked younger, she was the oldest child on the ship. The Jewish rescue committee in Britain sent her on to Glasgow to live with a Russian Jewish family. Two years later, unhappy with her adopted family, she embarked on a Japanese freighter bound from England for Shanghai. Because of a British-Chinese accord dating to the nineteenth century, Shanghai was an open city, a free port. Between 1938 and 1941, 18,000 Jews took refuge there.

The Japanese army had already taken possession of Shanghai in 1937, and in early 1943 they confined the Jews to a ghetto surrounded by barbed wire. Khema, who had a clerical job with an import-export business, could leave the ghetto for work; she and her parents lived in a two-room apartment on her meager income. They sold their remaining possessions, one by one, to pay for food. One day, while she stood on a street corner in the ghetto, an acquaintance near her was blown to smithereens by a bomb.

Ayya Khema's dear father died just five days before the war ended. Her mother remarried, and Khema herself married an older man. After the war, she worked as a secretary for the American army of occupation until, in 1949, she and her husband and two-year-old daughter emigrated to Los Angeles on the last transport ship to leave Shanghai before Mao Zedong's Red Army consolidated its control over all of mainland China.

Resettled in California, Khema worked for the Bank of America for ten years. She ended her marriage in 1960, taking her three-year-old son with her and leaving her thirteen-year-old daughter with her husband. She then went to live at a biogenic community founded by Dr. Edmund Szekely, just across the Mexican border from San Diego, that promoted organic foods and various spiritual teachings. There she became a vegetarian.

During this period, she also met and married a German engineer. They traveled through Mexico, Central America, and South America by jeep. Since the Pan-American Highway had not been completed, many rivers had no bridges and so had to be forded. The couple then emigrated to Australia, where they ran an organic farm in the 1960s. Khema was a proto-hippie, obviously a woman ahead of her time.

She began Buddhist meditation in the 1970s and, amazingly, taught herself the meditative absorptions (*jhanas*), a practice of deep concentration that was almost a lost teaching. Her second husband, seeing that she was more interested in meditation than marriage, left her in 1975. Four years later, she was ordained as the very first Theravadin female monk in a thousand years. After her ordination, she moved to Sri Lanka to study more closely with her preceptor—the monk who had sponsored her for ordination. She lived with breast cancer for the last fourteen years of her life. She died in 1997 on All Souls Day.

When Ayya Khema said, "Do the five daily reflections," even on videotape, she meant it. I did not question her wisdom.

These five reflections are nowadays called the

Heavenly Messengers because of a story told by the Buddha.

A previous Buddha lived a life of luxury, a very protected life, much as we Americans do today. In his late twenties, he asked his chauffeur (his chariot driver) to take him out to the city. That day, he saw, for the first time in his life, an old person. The next day, he saw a sick person. The third day, a corpse that lay by the side of the road. Here is that young man's response:

> While I had such power and good fortune, yet I thought, "When an ordinary person who is subject to aging sees another who is aged, he is shocked, humiliated, and disgusted. For he forgets that he himself is no exception. But I too am subject to aging, not safe from aging, and so it cannot befit me to be shocked, humiliated, and disgusted on seeing another who is aged."
>
> When I considered this, the vanity of youth entirely left me.

We too are sometimes shocked to see old people or disgusted to see them in nursing homes. *Eeewww.* Yet this is not a fitting response, knowing that we ourselves will, believe it or not, look very much like that aged person whom we wrinkle our nose at, or whom we today dismiss as being *old*. When we are young or youngish, we have the self-centeredness of believing that *we* are so ultra-modern, and that the old person is *so* behind the times.

Especially in our youth-worshipping culture we really have to work at counteracting our own vanity, which manifests as ageism.

The prince had the insight that he, too, would grow old, and thus the vanity of being young and handsome dropped away from him. Most of us, even in middle age, retain the vanity of a good-enough-looking body. We are humiliated and ashamed when the body betrays us by wrinkling, sagging, or getting middle-age spread. Some of us work out frantically to lose weight, or we Botox our faces, trying desperately to look younger than our years. Looking old is so *bad—what will other people think of us?* —and yet so natural.

To continue this story, the Buddha reported that, upon seeing a sick person, the prince thought:

> *When an ordinary person who is subject to sickness, not safe from sickness, sees another who is sick, she is shocked, humiliated, and disgusted, for she forgets that she herself is no exception. But I too am subject to sickness, not safe from sickness, so it cannot befit me to be shocked, humiliated, and disgusted on seeing another who is sick.*
>
> *When I considered this, the vanity of health entirely left me.*

I'll admit, I myself have the vanity of a healthy body and the pride of good health. Except for that little detail of cancer. Up to now, I haven't taken any daily medications.

But I was having my own close encounters with the Heavenly Messengers of aging and disease. And the thought of dying did occasionally wing into my mind.

I take a couple of multi-generational exercise classes, and when it comes time to do partner exercises, the young people don't choose me and my lumpy body with wrinkled skin. Occasionally, I have a teacher who teaches to the young bodies, leaving me to feel like a special-needs student who requires a lot of extra attention in order to attempt what the twenty- and thirty-somethings are doing so effortlessly. Without thinking about it, middle-aged people cling to the vanity of youthful bodies, and they prefer to be among their own kind, again without even examining their bias.

The Buddha-to-be then thought:

When an ordinary person, who is subject to death, sees another who is dead, he is shocked, humiliated, and disgusted, for he forgets that he is no exception. But I too am subject to death, not safe from death, so it cannot befit me to be shocked, humiliated, and disgusted on seeing another who is dead.

When I considered this, the vanity of life entirely left me.

I was very fortunate to be at my mother's bedside when she died and then to wash her body an hour later, when the hospice nurse arrived. Oh, how my mother loved her baths.

During her last day, she had a death rattle. My brother, Paul, said, "How can you stand to be in there with her?" I shrugged. She had seen Paul and me through years of asthmatic wheezing. The death rattle lasted only twelve hours. I was simply happy to be near my mother during her last hours on earth.

I have often heard people say, "I didn't go to see her because I want to remember her as she was." This phrase "I want to remember her as she was" is code for our disgust at death. We don't want to get too close to the dying; we don't want to look at the future that awaits our very own selves—death.

I was choosing not to be disgusted by aging, sickness, and death. I did not make them "other"—other than me, that is—an enemy. I was choosing to look closely and say "I too" am growing old, becoming diseased, and, yes, even dying, day by day.

There is a fourth heavenly messenger. On the fourth day, the prince left his palace with his chariot driver and saw a wandering ascetic in orange robes walking serenely down the street near an old person, a sick person, and a corpse. May I myself have that serenity, that equanimity.

These facts of life are called Heavenly Messengers. Every day we receive an invisible text message from our future. One of these days, I too will be wrinkled, or I too will develop a chronic disease, or I too won't remember where I left my glasses or my keys or my wallet. And I too will die.

We can look away and pretend we don't see. The

Buddha was from the warrior class; warriors are trained not to flinch. It was not "fitting" that he was shocked at the sights of aging, illness, and death. It's really not appropriate for us either, so we have to train ourselves to look these Heavenly Messengers square in the eye, instead of (a) pretending that we don't see them, or (b) believing that aging, illness, and death are not going to happen to *us*.

These Heavenly Messengers were feeling very personal to me just now. They were front and center during my self-retreat as I contemplated them every day. They were knocking on my front door, reminding me that the lease on my abode will be expiring someday. I have to admit, the old place does need a lot more maintenance nowadays. Fortunately, this cancer is not an eviction notice.

One of the insights I've had on this retreat is that my body is only loaned to me. I pay the "rent" by nourishing this body, which cannot really be called "mine." Food, whether it is animal, vegetable, or mineral, is itself made up of earth, water, air, and a mysterious life force we call "heat" or "fire." These "elements" are on loan to me for the short amount of time it takes the body to compost them into usable bits. Then the body "pays back" the loan of the elements via the back door of the body. The stardust from which I am made is loaned to me for a very short time and is eternally re-circulating. Every cell, they say, is replaced within seven years. Then, *poof!* Ashes to ashes, dust to dust, and there's nothing me or mine remaining in this impersonal collection. I never owned this abode, this body, in the first place.

The heavenly messenger of disease, of cancer, has cleared a veil from my eyes. I can see more clearly now, thanks to this tough-love message from the Heavenly Messengers.

Scars

I am of the nature to grow old.
Aging is inevitable.

TEN DAYS AFTER surgery, the steri-strip in my armpit came off during the gentle wash I gave to my underarm during my nightly shower. Wrapped in a towel, I lifted my right arm and looked in the bathroom mirror at the lymph node scar under my arm. Hmmm. Not bad. And they shaved my underarm too. Whoa! That hasn't happened for decades. I barely recognized that hairless armpit as mine.

The steri-strip on the right side of my right breast came off a week later, revealing a beautiful scar, barely visible. Short and narrow, slightly pink and shiny. I suddenly felt a great affection for my surgeon, Dr. Rosen, for giving me this "beauty mark."

Over the years, scars both outer and inner have accumulated all over my body. I could call my collection of scars "aging"—the chicken pox scar on my forehead, from age six; the three-inch appendectomy scar from 1957, when I was nine; the scar across the top of my foot from crashing my nine-year-old brother's go-cart in the dirt and weeds, when I was thirteen.

My right eardrum is scarred by too many earaches, too many burst eardrums as a child. Now, I hear less well out of that aging ear. I wouldn't be surprised if my lungs were scarred from all that childhood asthma, infection after infection for twelve years.

Last summer, I watched a mother tsk-tsk over a mosquito bite on her twelve-year-old daughter's face—a red bump marring the beautiful smooth young skin. The mother wanted to prevent any blemishes and save her child from any suffering.

I've collected all sorts of blemishes as I have aged— some visible, some not. No matter how wonderful a childhood is, everyone is damaged in some way or another. It's called *dukkha*. We all suffer. Scars, bother inner and outer, can be thought of as the record of the *dukkha* we have encountered in our lifetime.

I could consider my scars as badges of life, the idea of perfect skin having been lost a couple of decades ago, in my mid-forties, when the wrinkles set in. I have a smallpox vaccination scar on my upper left arm, from age fourteen (1962), and a scar on my upper right arm where a skin cancer was removed at age fifty-five. The skin cancer was a souvenir of visiting New Zealand, where there is a hole in the ozone layer.

The dermatologist zaps little squamous cells on my face every year, leaving small, pale marks, which I prefer to skin cancer.

The body ages; more marks. Now I have these two short scars from breast cancer.

The invisible inner scars are marked on my psyche; many of them are well healed over now. A depression after the breakup of my first romantic relationship—healed by meditation, though it took some additional years to regain my footing. Then fifteen years of a scab I kept picking at—*I am unlovable. No one wants me.* This invisible wound was healed in my early forties by Bill.

And now, with visible scars on my skin from breast cancer, I would say that my psyche is barely bruised by this event.

Health Insurance

I am of the nature to become ill.
Sickness is unavoidable.

T HE REASON I have health insurance is that I know
I am of the nature to become ill, and I don't want to
have to pay thousands of dollars for something I almost
take for granted—my health.

Health insurance is actually sickness insurance—
insuring myself against the expenses of future illness.
With the diagnosis of breast cancer, that future has
arrived. I can't even imagine how much all this is going
to cost.

Just a few years ago, I had a $10,000 deductible
because, I said, I did not want to have the stress of calling my health insurance provider, and perhaps arguing
with them, about paying my medical costs. Actually, I
was playing the roulette of self-insurance, and betting on
my continued good health. By saving myself $100–200
a month, *not* paid to BlueCross BlueShield, I thought
I could stand the risk of a high deductible. If I "saved"
$2,000 a year on my premium, in five years I would "earn"

the high deductible, which I would rather have in my pocket than theirs.

Since I turned sixty-five, Medicare and my supplemental insurance cover everything. Everything. No more 80/20 *meshugas*, no more co-pay. My deductible is a paltry $150, and that is covered by my supplement. I have loved Medicare since the moment I was covered.

One of the key decisions was to choose my first policy wisely. I was looking forward to sorting out my Medicare details with Norman, my dear friend and insurance agent. However, Norman dropped dead two weeks before his sixty-fifth birthday, so, two months before *my* sixty-fifth birthday, I called one of his co-workers.

When my friends start asking me about which Medicare plan to choose, I say, "Call an insurance agent." Of course, you want to call one whom a friend recommends to you—an agent who is looking out for your best interests and not his own.

Making the right choices of your Medicare plan, a supplemental plan, and a drug plan before your sixty-fifth birthday is the key to what comes next. This is not a time to gamble on your health, as I did in my early sixties, because when illness strikes, as it most certainly will, those co-pays, deductibles, and network providers will become burdensome to you.

Other friends have not been as fortunate in their Medicare choices as I have been. Changing their plans in midstream, once they have the diagnosis of cancer, is complicated and more expensive in the long run—and for one friend with prostate cancer, it has even delayed treatment.

Disease is unavoidable for the aging body and prone to be stressful enough, even before the bills come in. I feel extremely grateful to have a stress-free Medicare plan.

The Gift of Cancer

I am of the nature to die.
Death is unavoidable.

Ayya Khema instructed us to consider all the ways in which we might die, from best-case scenario to worst. I visualized myself dying on a warm day out in my garden, perhaps lying down on the ground, perhaps sitting in a lawn chair under an apple tree. (My best-case scenario.) I won't tell you my worst; you've seen enough movies that you can imagine your own worst-case scenario. But I did imagine myself on the side of a highway looking lovingly into some EMTs eyes as I breathed my unexpectedly last breath.

I imagine sudden death is quite a shock to the body-mind. Such a death usually results in a more difficult grief for the survivors. Given a choice between sudden death or having advance warning, which would you choose?

Many people want to die in their sleep, to be unconscious of death. I myself would choose having some notice, some time to prepare, some time to say good-bye. I would like to be conscious of dying. From this perspective, dying from cancer looks like a gift because it gives you time—two weeks or two months or two years—to prepare yourself and your loved ones.

Now I have a new scenario to imagine—dying from cancer. This too could go from best-case scenario—quick and pain-free—to the worst—a prolonged dying, which wears out everyone around me and is quite expensive. One way or another—fast or slow, easy or difficult—I too will die.

I *so* want to go easily and relatively quickly, yet I've seen friends and acquaintances linger for months, even years losing more and more mobility. I don't want to be a burden, but really, I have no say in that. I can write down my intentions, but who knows whether life will work out that way?

In the end, death is just another opportunity to surrender to Life, trusting that Life knows better than I do about how to die.

Impermanence

Everything I cherish will change and vanish.

ON THE DAY of my surgery, my sister sent me a big, full bouquet of magenta carnations and alstroemeria, generously filled in with unopened fragrant stargazer lilies and magenta mums. What a feast for the eyes. What a beautiful way to say *I love you*.

The bouquet continued to look fantastic for about ten days, and then the carnations looked decrepit. Out they went to the compost pile. Then the alstroemeria. The last lily bloomed and wilted, and then all that was left were the mums, which I grouped into three smaller vases. I cherished that bouquet, took photos of it, blogged about it, and bragged about it. But that cherished bouquet vanished bit by bit until, finally, it was gone, completely gone. I sent the beautiful wide-mouthed red vase to the hospice thrift store. Another thing, which I cherished for two weeks, vanished from my life.

One of these days, my nearest and dearest sister will vanish from my life. Knowing that our time is limited, I cherish my time with my sister, whom I visit in Idaho every year. Even though we may be doing nothing more than sitting companionably in her dark living room, drinking tea, and watching dawn slowly come to Lake Pend Oreille, this too will, one day, vanish from my life.

One of these days, I too will vanish from this world and be tossed onto the compost pile along with a bunch of wilted flowers.

Karma

Karma is the only thing I own.

IN TRUTH, KARMA is my only legacy. Though I spend a lot of mental energy arranging the material world by writing my will and my advance directives, by doing various forms of financial planning, and by writing one book after another, my only true legacy is my actions. The consequences of my actions accompany me wherever I go and ripple out in ways I cannot foresee.

I first realized the importance of karma at a seminar on Buddhist Psychology in 2000. As a result, I set about pruning the biggest weed in my mental garden—aversion. If you reap what you sow, as karma promises, why, oh why, had I spent the first fifty-two years of my life sowing the seeds of aversion? What had I been thinking? That I was going to right the wrongs of the world by being angry? Oh, how I love to push away the unpleasantnesses of life with an opinion, a judgment, a quick flick of the tongue. I could be a professional critic.

To prune this giant, overgrown weed in my psyche, I started with simply being mindful when irritation or frustration arose, as it did several times a day. I'd hold my horses, while mentally noting, "Irritation . . . Irritation" and feeling the *grrrrr* in my body—jaw set, teeth slightly clenched, eyes slightly tensed, breath shallow, and often my whole body awash with adrenalin, which gave me so much energy and felt great. I tried to put the brakes on my flippant opinions by zipping my lips. I stopped thinking *What's the matter with them? They're just weak if they can't take a harmless little jab.* I began to soften into how the "harmless little jab" felt to me. After about a year, I noticed that my good friends seemed to feel safer around me. Occasionally, I would be in a situation guaranteed to get a rise out of me, and no opinion would arise. Eventually, I began to laugh at things that previously would have set me off. *Oh, can you believe it? Ha!*

Later, I learned to avoid certain situations. On retreat, for instance, I sat with my back to the buffet table, because I didn't want to have an opinion about how much the fat guy put on his plate.

Karma means "action." When we've repeated an action often enough, it becomes a habit. So another word for karma is *habit*. Just what kind of habits do we want to cultivate? When Chogyam Trungpa Rinpoche was asked, "What is reborn?" he replied, "Our bad habits." I certainly don't want to be reborn (just in case that's a possibility) with the habit of irritation. I certainly don't want to feel irritated on my deathbed, unable to say a word, yet frustrated at someone or something. So I start my mind training now. Pause. Be mindful. Feel the irritation, the frustration, the impatience. Forgive myself for not understanding. Then replace the negative with the positive.

Loving-kindness and compassion are the antidotes to anger and aversion and all the members of the irritation family. First, I can have compassion for myself for trying to set things right so unskillfully. Have compassion for myself, who "inherited" aversion from my father, who inherited it from his father, et cetera. Have compassion for the person (me) who is slowly learning new habits of mind, and unlearning old habits, even if I have to relearn them every day for years.

Kindness begets kindness, and irritation begets irritation. The time to change my karma, change my habits of mind, is right now, with the next breath or the next thought. My actions, my speech, and especially my thoughts have consequences. How I act, what I say, what I think just digs that rut deeper. Let those actions, words, and thoughts spring from kindness toward all beings.

Today Is a Good Day to Die

I REMEMBER ONE PARTICULAR line from the movie *Little Big Man* (1970), a Western with many scenes depicting the Cheyenne nation in the mid-nineteenth century. Old Lodge Skins (played by Chief Dan George) tells his adopted white grandson, Little Big Man (played by Dustin Hoffman), "Today is a good day to die." Together they walk out to the prairie. Old Lodge Skins lies down in the grass, ready to die. Then it starts raining, so he trudges back to his tipi, saying, "Sometimes the magic works, and sometimes it doesn't." Again the next day he tries to die, and again he says, "Today is a good day to die."

In 1987, when I was researching my book *Following the Nez Perce Trail* at the age of thirty-nine, I was on the road for nine months, sleeping in my tent every night. Every morning I awoke with this prayer on my lips: "Today is a good day to die."

I was trying to feel my way into the poignant journey of the Nez Perce Indians in 1877 as they fled from the U.S. Army. Seven surprise attacks and several raids and skirmishes meant people were dying all along the 1,200-mile trip. Whether good or bad, any day could be a day to die, as hundreds of Nez Perce did.

This prayer is still with me when I read about a traffic accident or a war casualty. That person did not get up on that morning expecting that they would die today. Death can surprise us anytime. Perhaps it probably won't, but still, it might. We don't really know, and we have no say-so. Death is certain; the time of death is uncertain. We've all had enough close calls that we can feel grateful to our guardian angels who have kept us safe—so far.

We take on a reminder-of-death practice to acquaint ourselves with the facts of life. Slowly, ever so slowly, we desensitize ourselves to anxiety that stems from the fear of death, so that, one of these days, when we are face to face with Death, or with its cousin Cancer, we can honestly say, "Today is a good day to die."

Every day is a good day to die. And once we realize that, we will realize: not only is it a good day to die, it's a very good day to live.

Life's Lessons in Dying

HERE'S THE COURSE catalogue of my lessons in death and dying.

Death and Dying 101

- My grandfather died when I was twenty-eight. He was seventy-eight. Daddo was a physical fitness buff who ate health food in the 1950s. I last saw him do a handstand on his seventy-second birthday, the day Neil Armstrong walked on the moon.
- When I visited him in the ICU, he was in a coma due to congestive heart failure, and he moaned one syllable. The day before he died, I went into his room with Aunt Jenny, and Daddo moaned two syllables, as if to say "Jen-ny." That's how I realized that the comatose are still aware and can still hear.
- The morning he died, I woke up and wanted to go visit him, but my mother and aunt weren't going, so I didn't either. The phone call came an hour later, and that's when I felt the regret of not following my intuition.

Death and Dying 102

- *Mindfulness would be a really useful skill to have on my deathbed.*
- I had this insight as a result of my first ten-day retreat—a present to myself for my thirtieth birthday over the holidays of the New Year, 1978. Thus, I made the commitment to practice mindfulness.

Death and Dying 103

- *Today is a good day to die.*
- I practiced this prayer every day in 1987 while I was on the road and camping for seven months, researching the Nez Perce Trail.

Death and Dying 104

- My dear grandmother, Nonnie, died in November 1987. I was thirty-nine; she was eighty-four.
- I touched her hands as she lay in the coffin and was startled that her fingers were cold.

Death and Dying 201

- I took the hospice volunteer training when I was forty-five because I knew my parents wouldn't live forever. I wanted to be prepared when the time came.
- Although I didn't realize it then, my dad had just visited me for the last time.
- When I talked with friends who had taken the hospice training and whose parents had died, I heard all

the details, some of which inspired me, eventually, to think outside the box.

- I learned to simply listen and not to promote my own values in any way. I should not assume that I know what the dying person or their family needs. Ask. Communicate, even if I think the dying person is not awake or conscious. Be present.

Death and Dying 202

- My first hospice patient died on my forty-sixth birthday.
- He had told his wife that while he was sleeping, he was traveling to Taiwan and Japan, the other side of the world, where he had been stationed in the service three decades earlier. She took him seriously. I could imagine how a dying person has a foot in two worlds—our world and the other, unknown. A bardo, a between place.

Death and Dying 203

- I visited other hospice patients who died—one or two a year. Supporting their family members was as important as or, often, more important than my relationship to the patient.
- I realized that until the moment we die, we are all living people. And from the moment we're born, we're all dying people.

Death and Dying 301

- My father died in 1997; he was seventy-nine. I was forty-nine.
- My sister and I were with him for his last six days. She cooked; I did his dialysis exchanges. Brother Beau, who lived next door, took care of the paperwork.
- I had never imagined wanting to do personal care for a dying person, yet being that intimate with my father felt like a great gift.
- In the week before Dad died, he could still walk around and go to the bathroom himself, but he was having a bit of kidney-failure-induced dementia, which he did not like, not one little bit.

Death & Dying 302

- I was overcome by the sadness and knowledge that everything Dad did or said or we did or said was for the last time. It would never, ever happen again.
- The four of us children (all in our forties) hung around the living room. Dad was still in control of the television—a throwback to a familiar constellation of thirty years earlier.
- My dad was an authoritarian bully who scared the rest of us into submission. As he became weaker, I could dare to creep closer to him and remember the fun daddy whom I had loved so deeply when I was quite young.
- Walking through the doorway between his living room and his kitchen one day, I was struck by grace.

In that mystical moment, I knew there was nowhere on earth that I would rather be.

- Though I rationally knew my father would die within a few days, I watched my mind play tricks on me with "not yet" and "later" and "maybe he has another month." Denial is *so* deep and *so* strong.

- A few hours after he died, I found an empty bottle of sleeping pills on his bedside table. I couldn't make that suspicion make sense since I had talked to him half an hour before he died, but I wouldn't put it past him to hurry the dying process along.

Death and Dying 303

- I interviewed my father for an hour each morning for four mornings so that I could write his obituary. It was the first time I had heard the comprehensive story of his life.

- In effect, in just a few days I gave my siblings an intensive hospice volunteer training.

- We kept Dad's body at home for six hours. My brother and I dressed his body at the funeral home, which turned out to be quite funny. This enabled my brother and me to give dry-eyed eulogies at the funeral.

- The funeral was not about the dead body in the casket. It was an opportunity to be surrounded by people who had loved my dad.

- We handed out envelopes of Dad's hollyhock seeds to everyone. After everyone else had gone to the reception at the church, I alone watched the casket being lowered into the earth. I saw the dump truck dump the load of earth onto his casket. *Ker-thud.*

Death and Dying 304

- I got together a support group of hospice volunteers to read *A Year to Live* by Steven Levine during 1998, when I was fifty. We met monthly for three years.
- I love talking with fellow hospice volunteers, because everyone has done their work regarding death and dying by going through the hospice training, and we can talk about *anything* related to death in a matter-of-fact way, without cringing, without tiptoeing around the obvious, and without skittering off to a different subject.

Death and Dying 305

- As part of my Year to Live practice, I went to India when I was fifty-one and watched funeral pyres burning along the Ganges. I spent hours looking and watching as a meditation, as a contemplation, not as a voyeuristic sightseer.
- The men of the family carried the body on a stretcher and placed it on the stack of wood. The fire was lit, and, after a while, the body, the skeleton glowed before collapsing. The body turned to ashes before the very eyes of the family.
- In some pyres, where the family could not afford sufficient wood, legs and arms were sticking out of

the fire. The fire-tenders from the lowest caste raked up the limbs the way I rake branches into a burning brush pile. Eventually, they swept the cremains into the Ganges.

- These open-air cremations were a holy event. No photos!

Death and Dying 306

- I visited my dear Aunt Jenny, aged seventy, two weeks before she died in December 1999, and I told her how much I loved her.
- My cousins reported that her last word was "Mother!" I loved this vicarious glimpse of my grandmother, Nonnie.

Death and Dying 307

- My mother died three weeks after her sister, my Aunt Jenny, in January 2000. Mom's skin was yellow from cirrhosis. I was with her for her last eleven days, and when she died, I washed her body with the help of a hospice nurse. I was fifty-two years old; she was seventy-four.
- A year earlier, I had spent a month working on a eulogy for my alcoholic mother before I could say something true and kind.
- My mother was not ready to meet her Maker. She had been sober for her last month of life because she could no longer reach her bottle of vodka under her chair. She had many regrets.

- During her last twelve hours, I midwifed the difficult labor of her dying, until she was transfixed by the light outside her window. In the moment before her death, she seemed surprised. I hope it was a good surprise.

Death and Dying 308

- On every retreat for the next five or so years, my meditation would be "interrupted" by memories of my mother's and my father's deaths. This purifying process really cleaned out all the corners of grief till very little remained. As one meditation teacher says, "The mind is like a flooded basement. When you meditate, the water level goes down."

Death and Dying 401

- I practiced the five daily reflections every day for five years.
  I am of the nature to grow old.
  I am of the nature to become ill.
  I am of the nature to die.
  Everything I cherish will change and vanish.
  Karma is the only thing I own.

Death and Dying 402

- I visited one hospice patient for seven years, 2005–2012.
- As she neared the end of her life, I visited her in the ICU and whispered her favorite meditation, a body

scan, into her comatose ear. Her monitor began to beep warningly. The next morning, I did the same thing, and gave her "pointing-out" instructions.* "The body is just a bunch of twinkling lights in space. Why, looky there." She died forty minutes later.

- I wrote an article about this woman, "The Longest Hospice Patient," for the magazine *Tricycle: The Buddhist Review*. The editor took my 5,000 words of feeling and trimmed the piece to a cogent 2,000-word story.
- I received no response from readers.

Death and Dying 403

- I was diagnosed with breast cancer at the age of sixty-seven.
- I had known that I could see the horizon of my lifespan, but it suddenly felt very close.

---

* Pointing-out instructions point out the nature of mind, that all appearances arise within the mind, and thus that there is nothing *other* than mind. Yet mind itself is emptiness and openness beyond conceptualization.

Snow and Ice

THE WINTER OF my lumpectomy was brutal. Snow arrived the day before Thanksgiving and continued building up, so that by March 1 all the usual landmarks in the yard—lawn chairs, garden statues, fences—were buried under four feet of snow. The temperature dropped into the single digits in early January and stayed there into March. There was no January thaw, only more deep freezing.

The path between our house and The Sweet was the width of a snow shovel, with snow on both sides up to my chest. Every morning, the higher and warmer March sun melted the ice on the stone walkway, and every evening the meltwater that accumulated on the walk, with no place to go, refroze into a skating rink. Every day, I snow-shoveled the water off the walk, pitching it into a nearby snowbank.

The snow itself was frozen crusty, with nothing soft and fluffy about it. If I tried to walk on it, I sank in up to my waist and floundered. The accumulation of snow on the north side of the roof had turned into a two-foot-thick glacier—sixteen inches of snow on top of eight inches of ice.

We have double-entry back doors; we have to walk through the woodshed before entering the house. The icicles hanging from the beams of the woodshed might melt if the shed warmed up to thirty-three degrees, and then at night the meltwater on the plywood floor froze the beat-up old rugs in the shed into blocks of ice

In my thirty-five years of living in this house, I have never before had ice dams on the roof. Everyone was complaining of ice dams leaking water down the inside of their north walls; some people had ceilings that were peeling and suffering water damage. Everyone was chopping ice off the north side of their roof. So my work detail, in between meditations, was to set up the extension ladder in four feet of snow, angled against the low woodshed roof. Getting to the ladder was an exercise in swimming through snow. Bundled up to the gills in ten-degree weather, hammer in hand, I gleefully pounded away and caused avalanches off the roof, which fell only three feet to the pile of snow accumulating below the roofline. Pretty soon, the mound of avalanched snow and ice was higher than the roof.

I actually had fun clearing the snow off the walks and off the roof, but every winter one or two of my friends slip on the ice and break a wrist or a hip. A dusting of snow on top of ice is particularly treacherous. Every time I walked out the front door, I strapped Yaktrax or, my new favorite, Stableicers, on my boots. I used my hiking poles to walk down the road. I really tried to remember that I am a senior citizen and not to think of myself as a plastic-boned teenager. I am of the nature to have old bones, maybe brittle bones, that break.

The winter of my life is in the forecast. One of these days, my body will be snowed under. This year, I played in the snow and slid on the ice. Whee! But winter will win.

Insights

I PRACTICE INSIGHT MEDITATION, and on every retreat, a new insight comes to me. Usually, the longer the retreat, the deeper the insight. On my first ten-day retreat, I had the insight that mindfulness would be a very good skill to have on my deathbed.

When I tell my friends about an insight, like that one, it sounds banal, very commonplace. *Yeah, yeah, yeah,* they may think. They are receiving this insight with their minds, where it soon becomes lost among all the other "inspirational" passages they've ever read in their lives. "Mmm-hunh." *Yes, that's a good idea.* A good idea that is soon forgotten.

The thing about a true insight is that it is received in the heart, or maybe the whole body. Beginning meditators often say, "I feel so relaxed." Yes. That's what keeping your mind in the present moment does: it relaxes the body. Telling that insight to a friend elicits the same "unh-hunh." Or a "that's nice, dear" response. The listener receives the insight with her mind, not with her heart or body. The truth of our insights cannot really be conveyed in words. Justice may be blind, but truth is silent.

At the end of a retreat, the teacher usually says something like "Don't try to tell your friends about your retreat. If they ask, sum it up in a couple of sentences. If their eyes glaze over, stop talking. By all means, do not try to convert your parents."

My friends are usually content with my answer to their question "How was your retreat?" "Oh, good," I say. That's it. A few meditation friends may ask for a summary, so I will give them a paragraph.

As for my insights from my month-long retreat, one of them was: "Our bodies are on loan from Mother Nature. Everything is on loan. There's nothing personal about these bodies."

If I share this with someone, I might receive a nod of the head. Not a nod to say, *Brother, ain't that the truth! I know just what you're talking about.* But a nod to say, *Unh-hunh. I understand those words, but I don't really understand what she is saying. Oh, well. That's just Cheryl. She says the strangest things sometimes.*

My friends are my peers; I am not their spiritual teacher. So they think that what I am saying is just me saying some silly thing I sometimes say. An ordinary thing that friends say to friends. We're equals, after all. Aren't we? But we may not be equals in insight, equals in wisdom. So a nugget of gold is passed over as fool's gold.

As I go along in my practice, I become more open to the insights that friends tell me about. For instance, when my friend Debby says, "You know, Cheryl, thoughts really are homeless," I take this as a deep teaching, though

I have not seen this insight for myself, nor do I truly understand it.

Sometimes I borrow the insights of my teachers; I take their wisdom on faith, even though I haven't had those particular insights of impermanence or not-self myself.

The Buddha invites us to look deeply into the nature of life and to have our own insights. "See for yourself," he says. Nobody else can see it for you.

My body is on loan to me. Every day, I pay Mother Nature back and give "my" composted material to the earth, "my" air to the breeze, "my" water to the clouds, while the heat of the skin varies with the ambient temperature. "My" air is never mine, anyway. I'm often breathing other people's air. "My" 70-percent-water body is never "my" water. Water comes in the mouth door and leaves via the trap door at the bottom of the torso. Water in, water out. How could it ever be mine?

If you asked me, "Are you your body?" I would snort and say, "Of course not!" Yet when one thing goes wrong with the body—either something small like a cold, or something bigger, like cancer—I am suddenly clinging to "my" body with all my might. What happens there? I know very well that *I have a body, but I am not my body*, and yet I hang on to this body for dear life.

The ego doesn't want its vehicle to break down or rust with cancer or expire, because then our individuality wouldn't have a home. The ego needs the body to carry it around. The ego doesn't want cancer, doesn't want anything to mess around with the body that it inhabits. Yet the physical body is aging and dying from the minute it is born.

As I continue to explore and contemplate this sticky belief in "my body," an insight or several other mini-insights may arise, eventually relaxing my grip on "my body" as I come to a felt understanding of "I have a body, but I am not my body."

Many other insights have been lent to me by my Dharma friends and teachers. Now I freely offer you the loan of this insight: "My body is on loan to me. One day it will be time to pay back that loan in its entirety."

Oncotype DX

I WENT FOR MY follow-up appointment with Dr. Rosen, the surgeon, four weeks after my lumpectomy. Nan had had her follow-up appointment eight days after her surgery, but it's no use comparing my experience to hers. This was the way Life was unfolding. Wanting something different would be like pushing a river. Wanting something different would only exasperate me. That's useless.

There were reasons for the "delay," of course. Dr. Rosen was on a two-week skiing vacation. The week he returned, I was on a one-week retreat at Insight Meditation Society in Barre, Massachusetts. Yes, I could have taken half a day to drive to Brattleboro, have my appointment, and then return to the retreat; but during that first month after the surgery I was in a holding pattern anyway, waiting to heal.

I took my nurse-friend Barbara with me to see Dr. Rosen. Dr. Rosen recommended the Oncotype DX test to me. "But only if you're willing to entertain the possibility of chemotherapy," he said. "If you have a high score, then you'll need chemotherapy. If you already know you don't want to do chemotherapy, then the test is useless." They send off a sample of my tumor tissue and test it for twenty-one genes. Usually, the oncologist orders this test, but Brattleboro is a small town with a small hospital, so Dr. Rosen ordered the test for me in order to save some time and save me an extra visit to the oncologist. "It will take two and a half or three weeks for the results to come back," he said.

As I left his office, the receptionist made my appointment with the oncologist for me. "Who do you want?" she asked. "Mills or Nickerson?" All my women friends went to Letha Mills. "She's only here on Wednesdays, so you can see her on April 22."

Another month to see the oncologist? Oh no. What had happened to my streak of good luck? I knew from my neighbor that Dr. Mills, age sixty, was about to get married, and she'd be on her honeymoon for three weeks. Oh, brother, I seemed to be running into doctors' vacation schedules.

During the next twenty-four hours, I sent e-mails to Barbara, brainstorming various possibilities. Should I try to get in earlier with Dr. Nickerson? Should I use one of the oncologists in Keene? Was I establishing a lifelong relationship here? Should I try Dartmouth-Hitchcock, the teaching hospital? But I didn't want to be driving an hour and a quarter up to Lebanon, New Hampshire, every three months for the rest of my life.

Before I could settle on any of these suboptimal options, I received a call from Dr. Mills' office. "Dr. Mills has added one day to her schedule. Can you come in on April 6?"

"Yes!" I was desperate. Monday, April 6, fitted

perfectly into my schedule. I would be returning from my final weeklong retreat on April 4.

Then I had second thoughts. The results of my Oncotype DX test probably wouldn't be back until April 9 or 10. Oh, dear.

I called Dr. Mills' office and asked to speak with Agnes, the nurse practitioner. The surgeon had called Agnes the "chief cook and bottle-washer" of the oncology department. I had heard about Agnes for twenty years. She was a caring, do-everything, know-everything person on whom patients could depend

"Hi Agnes, you haven't met me yet. I have my intake appointment with Dr. Mills on April 6, but my Oncotype DX test results won't be back until later in the week."

"Oh, that's fine," Agnes said. "We're not Dana Farber. We don't have to have all the cards on the table, all the test results in, before we see you. Come on in. You never know, the test results might be back by then."

Music to my ears. Yes. This was just the kind of doctor's office I wanted to go to. I felt so lucky. I let go of useless worry and anxiety about the unknowable future of my treatment. No one, and I mean *no one* in the whole world, really knew what the next step of my treatment would be. Sure, the oncologist could make her educated guesses. Me trying to out-think the process would be a useless exercise. One day, one moment at a time, I thought. I have an appointment, and *che sarà, sarà*.

Now that that was settled, I could go to my weeklong retreat at the Barre Center for Buddhist Studies, the final week of my month of retreat, with a peaceful mind.

Do I Really Need the Oncotype DX?

THE DAY AFTER my appointment with Dr. Rosen, I started wondering why I even needed the Oncotype DX test. Clear lymph nodes, clear margins, and an in-situ cancer. It hadn't broken through the cell walls. All good news. Wasn't I done? I called Dr. Rosen.

"Why do I need the Oncotype DX test?" I asked.

"You have invasive cancer," he said.

I do? I thought "in situ" was not invasive.

"Okay, thanks," I said, and hung up.

I couldn't make his answer make sense, but I decided to trust Dr. Rosen's recommendation. *I'm going with his intuition*, I reasoned to myself. He has years of experience. He probably just "knows," even without some of the knowledge being rational. He probably just feels the answer.

This is what trust feels like—stepping forward into the unknown, even though it doesn't make sense, even though I don't or can't know. I love to know. I adore knowing things. The unknown is a foreign territory that I conquer with knowledge. But, just as when I was learning to walk the tightrope at circus school (three feet off the ground), the coach is right there, spotting me, as I focus on my end goal—the end of my walk on the tightwire. I *can* walk there, even without my usual supports of standing on a floor or understanding exactly what's going on.

I decided not to overthink my response about the diagnostic test. I decided to simply trust the surgeon. After all, his wife had had breast cancer recently. I would follow his lead. I majored in engineering in college. I can be curious. What would the gene test show? I was sure I would have a low score.

I e-mailed Barbara for her opinion. She thought I might as well continue; what did I have to lose? Barbara's a natural scientist; she's always curious; she's an excellent observer of the natural world; and she's methodical. Okay, coach. I'm trusting you.

Letha

BILL HAD NOT gone to any of my appointments with the surgeon, so he really wanted to go with me to my first appointment with the oncologist. The question in my mind was: *Chemotherapy? Or no chemotherapy?* The answer lay in the results of the Oncotype DX test, which had in fact arrived that morning. *Oh, Life! I love you. You are so good to me.*

As we sat in the waiting room, I was trying to divine the answer from what Nurse Navigator Kelly said as she walked through the waiting room, or from how Maureen, the receptionist, shuffled her papers. Bill was confident that my number would be low.

I picked up a peppermint Life Saver from the bowl on the end table that held magazines that I was too restless to read. If the answer was chemotherapy, I was ready to proceed. If the answer was no chemotherapy, I would feel relieved. As usual, my mind wanted to know the answer *right now* that it could not know for ten or fifteen more minutes.

If your score on the Oncotype DX test is less than 18, you have a low chance of recurrence. You might not even need radiation. If it's more than 31, you have a high chance of recurrence. Over 31 means you are definitely headed to chemotherapy. My score was 24, smack dab in the middle. There it was in large print: 15 percent. "You have a 15 percent chance of recurrence," said Dr. Mills, "if you take tamoxifen for five years."

Fifteen percent chance of recurrence means 85 percent chance of non-recurrence, and that sounded good enough to me. Although as Dr. Rosen, the surgeon, had said, "If you're in the 15 percent, then your chance of recurrence is 100 percent." Point taken.

"The research has been done with tamoxifen," continued Dr. Mills, "but that's the drug for premenopausal women. I'll probably recommend an estrogen inhibitor, Arimidex, for you. It's for postmenopausal women."

Then Dr. Mills told me a story. "Early in my practice," she said, "I recommended chemotherapy to a seventy-two-year-old woman. The chemotherapy threw her into old, old age, from which she never recovered."

I felt that what Dr. Mills was really saying was, "Since your score is in the middle, you're almost too old for chemotherapy unless you really, really need it." I could see from the explanation that I could lower my chance of recurrence from 15 down to 12 percent with chemotherapy. On the other hand, the risks of chemotherapy might be more than 3 percent at my age. Risk outweighing benefit means no chemotherapy. I breathed a sigh of relief.

I felt so grateful to the millions of women who had gone before me, and the thousands of women who had participated in studies that could be synthesized onto a single sheet of paper showing that, due to my particular combination of genes, I had a 15 percent chance of recurrence. This process has been so refined compared to twenty years ago, when the answer to all breast cancer was mastectomy. Since 2004 the Oncotype DX has been used to test your genes, and therein lies the answer, with guidelines for your personal remedy. Oncotype DX diagnoses your type of cancer genes.

Thanks to the decades and brigades of pink-ribboned women, I can have confidence in my treatment and feel in the pink myself.

I sucked in the fresh taste of that peppermint Life Saver.

PRO-ACTIVITY:
Radiation

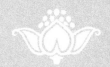

They Said "No" to Radiation

AFTER THE END of my five-week retreat in March, I could return to my regularly scheduled programs in April. I do like to have a weekly massage, and I try to schedule it for the day after my circus classes. Flexibility 101 is a workout for the hips, and Trapeze 101 is a workout for the shoulders, but then I need a massage to work out the kinks.

While I was under the merciful hands of Kathryn, the masseuse, she told me about a new chiropractor in my old chiropractor's office. My chiropractor, Catherine, was unable to come into the office because her breast cancer of seven years previously had metastasized. She was now practically bedridden.

Two days later, I heard about another chiropractor I used to go to, twenty years ago. Her breast cancer had also metastasized. She, too, was not working. Neither of these women had had radiation. I could only guess what course of alternative treatments each one had decided on, since the grapevine was a bit thin on the particulars.

My heart sank. I hadn't thought about not doing

radiation. I had doubted something else (that I had invasive cancer and needed the Oncotype DX test), but I had not doubted radiation.

When I told the oncologist that I was surrendering to Life, she seemed surprised that I was saying yes to radiation. She must see patients who say no to her recommendations—chemo or radiation or drugs. There are women who want to choose their own treatment and follow their own sense of what is right for them.

Doubt is the opposite of trust, the opposite of faith. I had placed myself on the treatment conveyor belt, and I was surrendering myself to many highly-educated, highly experienced medical professionals. Of course, I could step off my treatment walkway at any moment, but I was having a hard time understanding why I might feel so strongly about my treatment plan that I would refuse radiation.

Can you see it creeping in? My desire to fix-it? My heart aches for the two chiropractors—one of them a daughter of my previous chiropractor, and the other a natural healer with highly developed intuition who had founded the Cornucopia Choice Holistic Health Center, which has two dozen alternative practitioners under one roof. In order to stop my heartache, my mind wanted to go to problem solving, and from there, it is a very short step to unsolicited advice. Even though both women were home-bound, and I had no chance of seeing them, that didn't stop my mind from going down the if-only-they'd-had-radiation road and giving them each a piece of my mind.

Stop, Cheryl. True compassion is a combination of caring and bearing. Caring—yes, of course. Instead of side-stepping the pain of I-don't-want-them-to-die, I can bear that pain, just as it is, and, in my imagination, send healing thoughts to each of them, just as they are.[*] Caring and bearing is the path to true peace of mind.

---

[*] Catherine died three months later.

Being Mortal

I N T H E D A Y S after my diagnosis, I read *Being Mortal* by Atul Gawande, a surgeon in Boston. This book was highly recommended by my neighbor.

I was having my own strong dose of mortality. No longer could I pretend that things were going to go on as usual. No longer could I take for granted "see you next time" or "see you next year." Maybe yes, maybe even probably yes, but maybe not.

I sent an e-mail to the hospice volunteer coordinator about what a great book *Being Mortal* is. She agreed, and I blithely replied, "Let's have a book discussion group on it. Maybe meet for four sessions and read two chapters a week." She agreed to do the publicity. I would facilitate the discussion group in April after returning from my five-week retreat. In fact, we'd start the day after I met my oncologist for the first time. That seemed very appropriate, perhaps because my oncologist's first name is Letha, which sounds like "lethal," and I was face to face with the lethality, the mortality of life.

Gawande, who is an excellent writer, articulated several points in his book about which I already had a gut feeling. He gave me the words to speak clearly about many of the issues that go along with aging, disease, and dying.

It used to be that people declined suddenly, and the family doctor, making a house call, knew where this body was going. Nowadays, people decline bit by bit, decline and recover not quite everything, decline like a river that pools and drops, pools and drops, never, of course, regaining its original elevation. Technology has blurred the lines between living and dying. With the aid of surgical and bionic interventions, life can be extended and extended and . . .

Where would you draw your personal line between *quantity* of life and *quality* of life? If you, like I, aim toward quality rather than quantity, then the time to have these what-to-do-when-I'm-nearing-the-end-of life conversations is now. A good place to start is "What makes my life worth living?" The answer will change as time goes on; possibly it will change every year. Right now, my answer includes "gardening." When I am no longer able to sit in the garden or enjoy a houseplant, then it's time to breathe my last breath of fresh air, even if that is a belabored, oxygen-scarce breath.

I also love my mind. I've told my durable power of attorney for health care that if I lose my marbles not to give me any antibiotics. Don't save my body if my mind isn't working.

The author spends three chapters on new designs for nursing homes, which, he points out, are currently designed to suit the patients' adult children, not the aged residents themselves. The children of the elderly want them to be safe; the elderly want their autonomy. Maggie Kuhn was right when she called retirement communities "glorified playpens where wrinkled babies can be safe and out of the way." During one session, I led a guided meditation about living in a local nursing home with a roommate. Oooh, that was an unpleasant future to imagine, even in the best "home," which, of course, never feels like home.

As for coping with the medical establishment to achieve your goal of quality of life, Gawande talks about three kinds of doctors: Doctor God knows everything, while Doctor Informative tells you all the background information in multisyllabic words you never heard before and can't remember now. I thought of my surgeon, who was a veritable fountain of information and research studies.

The doctor for the new millennium is Doctor Ask-Tell-Ask. In other words, the doctor we want for our old age spends more time listening than talking. Our gerontology doctor doesn't jump in with the fixes for our body's failing systems. The new old-age doctor will make sure we are as comfortable as we can be in our old, failing bodies without going to extreme measures.

Counterintuitively, hospice patients on palliative or comfort care can live longer than people with similar diagnoses who pursue aggressive treatment. One reason for this is that the hospice nurse is visiting the patient at home or in a dedicated hospice facility. When something goes wrong, the family calls hospice instead of 911. Therefore, hospice patients use the emergency room much less frequently. They stop aggressive treatments in favor of palliative care. And they actually take fewer pills, because preventative medication is stopped, and pills are limited to comfort care meds.

I need to have my advance directives in place. LaCrosse, Wisconsin, has been working at this for thirty years, and 96 percent of the residents have advance directives. Although 30 percent of Brattleboro residents report having advance directives, only 3 percent are registered with the state registry.

I want to make electronic copies of my advance directives and upload them to the national registry. Then, if they find me lying on the side of the road, the EMTs can look at my iPhone and find my instructions.

As I've already made clear, while I'm not quite ready to have DNR (Do Not Resuscitate) tattooed on my chest, I am seriously thinking about the tattoo AND (Allow Natural Death), which would enable my body to speak even when I cannot. I've written down my endgame wishes.* Since I am a child-free woman, I am just going to have to trust to the kindness of strangers for my care.

One participant in the book group was quite confident that baby boomers will change the aging game and, she hopes, the aging floorplan, during the next two decades. Someone else called this book "a game changer."

---

* See "In Conclusion" in *Lost, but Found* (2014).

I find myself referring to this book in casual conversation once or twice a week. The more we talk about the stuff, the better we all will be.

I love this book, because it popularizes the Heavenly Messengers of aging, illness, and death. *Being Mortal* gives us a context in which to speak of the unspeakables. I watched the PBS *Frontline* program featuring Atul Gawande and could see situations in which one spouse clearly did not want to speak of impending death, but instead kept talking about "when things get better."

I feel fortunate that Bill and I have some aspect of this mortality conversation at least once a week. "After I'm gone, Bill, are you going to . . . ?" I assume that he will move into town and find a new companion within a few months. He should have enough income to afford to rent a nice place in downtown Brattleboro. We're getting too old to own a house. And if Bill goes first, how am I going to maintain this house? Bill points this out every time he feels I'm not carrying my share of the load. "What are you going to do without me, Cheryl?" Good question.

Just the other day, Bill said, "We probably have fewer than ten years left to live in this house." He's right. Recognizing our own mortality as well as the limited lifespan of our home together makes every day with Bill at home in our home all the sweeter.

My Legacy #2

URING THE BOOM of the early part of the millennium, I was a philanthropist. With the help of a philanthropic adviser, I developed a mission statement, prioritized my interests, and developed an annual budget for charitable gifts. Although I wasn't a member of Bolder Giving, a nonprofit organization that offers peer support for generosity involving spectacular sums of money, I did seriously take to heart their message of giving away half of my assets. Why would I do that, you ask. All my nieces and nephews and stepchildren are well provided for. There is such a thing as leaving adult children too much money, which can easily lead to grandchildren with an unhealthy sense of entitlement. That's probably not what you had in mind for those dear souls.

My friend Samantha, a screenwriter, is always interested in what really motivates people, and she asked me, "If I stuck a fork in your arm and told you that you have to leave money to a person, who would it be?"

"You'd just have to kill me with the fork," I said. "I guess I'm a socialist at heart." Sharing the common wealth and aiming toward a moral economy has always made so much more sense to me than subsidizing white privilege and boosting one of my relatives into the upper middle class.

Money saps vigor; inheriting money certainly sapped mine. Leaving money to children and relatives is usually an emotional gift, not a rational gift. Money and love are often conflated. As my neighbor Whit asked, "Will they love you more if you give them money? Will they love you less if you don't?" (And if those are true, then is that "love"?) We want our relatives to love us, to remember us fondly. We also want *our* clan (read: our genes) to survive at any cost. Family, for most people, is part of their immortality project.

The financial meltdown of 2008 took the wind out of my philanthropic sails. Nevertheless, I continue to give away 90 percent of my now-lowered income every year. Of course, this generosity eats into my assets, but I do not want to be managing money in my old age, nor do I want to be scammed when I become vulnerable. How much money does an old lady (as I will be one day) actually "need," anyway?

I review my charitable plan annually, sometimes paying more attention, sometimes less. This year was a time to pay more attention. What was really most important to me?

First, making sure that Bill is well cared for, in the event that I die before he does. I want to leave him enough to maintain our house or to rent a nice place in downtown Brattleboro. For this eventuality, I really like the vehicle of the charitable gift annuity (CGA). These annuities provide me with an annual income for now, and that will shift to Bill when I die. When he dies, the gift (the remainder) goes to the charity I have designated.

All the conservation organizations are well set up and provide easy accessibility. Just send them the money, sign a piece of paper, and you're done. However, as much as I like the Sierra Club, the Nature Conservancy, the National Parks Foundation, etc., conservation and protecting the environment are not my highest priorities. For the past fifteen years, my mission has been to empower women to make wise choices about their lives. Once I defined that, many possibilities began to fall into place, and I saw that many other wonderful projects simply are not congruent with my personal mission.

I love micro-finance, which usually serves women in small villages in the Third World. Only a few micro-finance organizations offer the charitable gift annuities, and many organizations are so small that they cannot afford to.

So here I was, trying to figure out a way to set up CGAs for some small organizations that serve my mission of empowering women. I had left this mystery unsolved a few years before, and now it was time to figure it out.

My highest priority is women's organizations in general, and Buddhist women's groups in particular. A few years ago, I wanted to set up a CGA for the Alliance for Bhikkhunis, based in Santa Barbara. I called the Santa Barbara Community Foundation, and they said, "We only offer charitable gift annuities to residents of

Santa Barbara." *Are you kidding me?* Now, how to solve this problem . . . ?

I wanted to set up a CGA for the bhikkhunis at the Saranaloka Foundation in Placerville, California, but the community foundation there said, "We're not offering CGAs anymore, because they're not worth it. People are outliving their annuities." *Are you kidding me? You're in charge of setting these things up; I'm sure you can arrange the details to make it worth your while.* So now what? Leaving a legacy to Buddhist women is proving rather difficult.

Another type of gift I like to make is offering scholarships. I've set up college funds for my grandchildren. My sister and I set up the Wilfong Family Scholarship for the high school we graduated from, out in the Hoosier cornfields. My brother set up a scholarship in my mother's name at Greenfield High School in Indiana, the school she graduated from. This scholarship is set to be spent down to zero, but how do I feel about that? Having a little scholarship named after my mother provides her with a teensy bit of immortality. Am I willing to let her name die? Or would bumping the scholarship up to the minimum amount be a way to offer a legacy in my mother's name?

These and other questions do not have easy answers. They require contemplation to feel how this possibility or that resonates with my mission, my purpose, and my heart. This means keeping at it, not letting this or that question fall off my radar screen.

Maybe I have time to put off these decisions and wait for another day or some other year. Or maybe not.

Fred-the-Fungus

A YEAR AGO, MY neighbor Connie finally received a diagnosis for her daily headaches: she had a fungal mass growing in her sinus. She named it Fred-the-Fungus. The sinus that Fred was growing in was not one of the usual sinuses we think of, above the eyebrows or below the eyes. Rather, Fred was growing in the sphenoid sinus, behind the nose and behind the eyes, right next door to the brain.

After telling her friends about Fred, Connie adopted the policy of never speaking about the fungus again, unless someone asked. In other words, Fred did not become part of her daily or regular "organ recital," which we are all familiar with because so many of our friends recite the latest news about their current personal organ-in-distress.

Eventually, Connie went to the sinus clinic in Boston, and Fred was removed without incident.

After I went public with breast cancer, I decided to adopt Connie's "Fred policy." I didn't talk or overtalk about my diagnosis nor all the surgical details nor the ups and downs of treatment. But if someone asked, I was happy to share.

There were times, mostly in circus classes, where I

did refer to what was going on with my body. Class often starts with the coach asking, "Is there anything about your body I should know this week?"

"Here's my lumpectomy scar," I said as I pulled down the armhole of my tank top to reveal the pink incision. "And here in my underarm is the lymph node scar. The surgeon said exercise would be good for me." (I'm not sure he realized that I would be pulling myself up onto a trapeze bar.)

I might mention the most recent step in the process to my close friends. I blogged about the process and shared that on Facebook, in the name of educating the public and demystifying the specter of cancer.

People I met on the street, in the parking lot, or in the food co-op were often caring and concerned. Some were worried about me. I thanked each one for her thoughts. Some friends didn't mention it all, and neither did I. I've heard too many people complain about their complaints. I didn't want to be one of them.

What are we doing when we talk about our particular version of the aging body? Partly we are saying, *It didn't use to be like this. Where's that easy body that performed without a second thought?* Our engine and perhaps our energy is clunking and pinging; we can't accelerate as we used to. Our body has rust spots. We are having a direct experience of aging, illness, and, yes, even the mini-deaths of various body parts that we can live without. These are deep spiritual lessons that we resist. The body is deteriorating before our very eyes, but we don't want to see what that means. The failing body is a fascinating mystery—each one different, though there are similarities. So we talk about our heart, our blood pressure, our diabetes as if they are our darling, though naughty, children, our favorite topics of conversation.

If we see our illness, our chronic disease, as a problem—*It shouldn't be like this* or *This shouldn't be happening to me*—we want friends to commiserate with us. "Ain't it awful!" To commiserate is to share someone's misery or suffering, which means you share their stressful thinking. In contrast, compassion *feels* in sympathy with someone. Compassion has enough equanimity in it not to believe the stressful thoughts, but simply feels the distressed emotion without judgment. As I have said elsewhere, commiseration is counterfeit compassion.

Our first order of business is to be compassionate toward ourselves. One of the ways in which I like to practice self-compassion is to start with the contemplation that "I am of the nature to become ill. Sickness is inevitable." And then I begin to list dear family and friends who have also suffered from some aspect of disease. "Just like my father, I, too, am of the nature to have a chronic disease. Just like my mother, I too, am of the nature to be sick. Just like my dear friend, I, too, am of the nature to have cancer." I continue remembering friends, neighbors, people I don't know except by sight, difficult people, and people in my community. I am not exempt from this aging-and-disease process, which affects everyone. As I begin to see this more clearly, I become more equanimous with things as they are, more balanced with this disease as it is.

Once I become even slightly comfortable in my own skin about what's happening to this body as natural consequence of my *having* a body, I can relax a bit. I don't need to talk about my version of Fred. I can surrender to Life one more time.

No Sugar

AFTER MY RETREAT, I only read a couple of books about the anti-cancer diet. Although there are all kinds of course corrections I could make to my already dairy-free, gluten-free diet, in the name of ease of eating, I have committed to only one: no sugar.

Sugar feeds cancer, so say the Europeans, though American studies do not prove the link. Whatever the scientific quibbling on each side of the issue might be, I don't believe sugar can be good for us, or even acceptable. Sugar feeds fat and feeds lurking diabetes. Sugar used to be considered a medicine, and it really does help the medicine go down by blocking pain. Nowadays, though, sugar and, even worse, high-fructose corn syrup (the corn has been genetically modified), are hiding in every processed food.

Even as I say "no sugar," you already know that I've got to be kidding. Sugar is hiding in everything. I am not going to be a sugar Nazi. I will continue to eat crackers and tortilla chips. I will continue to eat mayonnaise on my tomato sandwiches. I will continue to eat my homemade granola with its half-cup of maple syrup spread over thirteen cups of oats, coconut, pumpkin seeds, almonds, walnuts, sesame seeds, hemp seed, flax seed, and chia seeds. What I really mean when I say "no sugar" is "no desserts."

No desserts is a plan that I have wanted to commit to for a long time. I'm not that fond of sweet things to begin with. I don't really like cakes or pies, though pie-eater Bill offers me a piece of his apple pie almost every night after dinner. I've stopped saying "Too sweet" to my sweetie. Instead, I say, "No thanks."

I'm not really interested in cookies (too sweet!) except for chocolate-chip cookies. Chocolate chips are my downfall. So when I say "no sugar" and "no desserts," I'm really saying "no chocolate-chip cookies."

I was on a no-sugar diet thirty years ago, in my mid-thirties. After three years, though, I slowly drifted into chocolate-chip cookies. I began to eat birthday cake at birthday parties with the subterranean thought that I didn't want to hurt the hostess's feelings by not eating the cake she offered, usually special-ordered from Hannaford supermarket. Or that flourless chocolate cake from Amy's Bakery downtown. Now, that cake was to die for. On second thought, maybe it's not worth dying for.

"No sugar" means not sharing a dessert when Bill and I go out to dinner. He's on his own with a slice of key lime pie (always too sweet anyway) or the triple-fudge chocolate cake (too much chocolate!). Usually, he wants to order a dessert, like flan, that I'm not interested in anyway; now he has free rein.

At the intermissions of plays or concerts, I try not to

go near the table with the home-baked goodies. Those goodies may be good for someone else, but they are not good for me.

No sugar means I'm not baking any more blond brownies, loaded with bittersweet chocolate chips and walnuts and an excellent way to use the grated summer squash in the freezer. No sugar means no rhubarb squares. I haven't come to peace with no rhubarb yet. Maybe I'll use stevia.

I now pay attention to the glycemic index of sweeteners. Glucose (aka dextrose) is 100—the base line. Sucrose or table sugar is 65; maple syrup, 54; honey, 50; fructose, 25; agave, 15. Stevia and the artificial sweeteners are zero, and thus are perfectly acceptable, though I find the taste of aspartame, cyclamate, and the like repellent.

Bittersweet chocolate, especially over 85 percent cocoa, is actually good for you, and it has very little sugar. After my surgery, one of my neighbors brought me a Green & Black chocolate bar—88 percent. I take this extra-dark chocolate with me on retreat to wake me up in the afternoon sits. Recently, visiting my sister, I left an 88 percent chocolate bar on the island in the kitchen. Her nearly-diabetic husband is having a hard time with his no-sugar diet because he definitely has a sweet tooth. "Arrghh," he said, taking a bite of the tempting chocolate bar. "It's not sweet."

"That's the point," I said.

The Sanskrit word for happiness or pleasure or sweet is *sukha*, which sounds temptingly like the word "sugar," though they are unrelated. The Dhammapada says, "If by renouncing a lesser happiness one may realize a greater happiness, let the wise woman renounce the lesser, having regard for the greater."[*]

I suppose this is what dieting tempts us with. We can have the greater happiness of a slim and trim body, if we would only give up the lesser happiness of eating too much.

A few of my friends find this easy when it comes to their diet. Josephine, a yoga teacher, eats only healthy foods. My sweetie, Bill, loves broccoli, I suspect, because he knows it's good for him, not because he actually loves the taste of it. I do accuse him of having all his taste buds in his ears, since he's not really interested in how food tastes.

But the lesser happiness often wins out. The diabetic has a hard time giving up sugar. An alcoholic finds it nearly impossible to give up alcohol. It breaks my heart to watch dear friends and family members choose substances that aren't good for them.

Can I give up the lesser happiness of sugar for the greater happiness of no cancer?

Refraining from sugar is like going on the wagon. It's a one-day-at-a-time thing. I still crave an after-dinner sweet, so I take a chewable vitamin C, which tastes like a SweeTart candy. Yes, it contains dextrose and fructose—two grams. At other times, for dessert I'll have a bowl

---

[*] Verse 290.

of my homemade granola with unsweetened hemp milk (chock-full of omega-3s) or homemade applesauce from the wild apple trees in my backyard.

It's time to focus on fresh-fruit sugars in my new diet. I love all the berries that are available from June through October, and Vermont apples during the winter. I want to feed my body healthy food, and I do not want to feed any stray cancer cells.

So, sweetie, no sweets for me.

The Anti-Cancer Diet
for the Mind

J UST AS IMPORTANT as the food I feed my body is
the food I feed my mind. Though it's not too difficult
to commit to a healthy diet now that I have cancer to
scare me into it, it's been a rockier ride to just say no to
my biggest stressor of all—a relationship with a certain
relative.

Resentment is as deadly as secondhand smoke and
junk food. Why would I want to feed my mind hostility
and ill-will? Because I want to be right?

Wake up, Cheryl. It's time to let go. Release your
grasp on this useless wanting the relationship to be different from what it is. You know how to let go. You've
done it before.

Well, yes, I have said "no" a few times to stressful jobs.
I come to the point, to the realization, that *it's time for me
to leave this job*. The job used to be fun, but now it isn't.
Or I've been passed over for raises or advancement. Or
I've gotten so irritated at the higher-ups that I've become
brittle. Or I think my supervisor is inept. Then it's time
to leave. Stewing in bitterness is not worth the trouble.

Instead of insisting that "they" change, I'm the one who needs to make a change—in employment.

I was seldom the one to say "no" to relationships with men, though I did with a few. More often, much more often, I was the one who was left. Usually what I then needed is what I call a psychic cut, which I tried to practice with ex-lovers. A psychic cut means no contact at all, because any contact at all kept my heart open to them and therefore unavailable to me or others.

In my thirties, I was entirely capable of carrying on phantom relationships for months. When I finally, actually talked to Ron, nine months after our one and only date, and he said, "Let's be friends," I knew that "friends" meant he didn't want to hurt my feelings, but that he didn't ever want to see me again. I gently closed the door in my heart to him, and a week later met my soul mate. Life usually hasn't opened the next door until I've closed that previous door good and tight.

There are friends and family members I have consciously drifted away from. I stop calling. Or I stop sending Christmas cards. If they're not interested or thoughtful enough to do some relationship maintenance, then I will just have to love them from afar.

One or two of my blood relatives drive me nuts. Yes, we are related, and I would like a real relationship, a good relationship, but is all the psychic work I put into it worth it? Maybe it's time to stop beating a dead horse. Maybe it's time to stop pretending that I like this person.

My biggest stressor is a relative. I will leave it at that,

and let you fill in the blank with your own relative who makes you want to pull out your hair or give that adult a good shaking. Here's my simple definition of *family*: they're caring, they're appreciative, and they create a sense of belonging. I grade my stressful relationship accordingly: Do I feel cared about? Do I feel appreciated? Do I have a sense of belonging with them? I do realize that if my stressor were grading me on the same criteria, I, too, would fail in caring, appreciation, and sense of belonging.

Research shows that couples who have long-lasting relationships give a lot of positive feedback to each other. There needs to be at least three positive interactions, and preferably five, for each negative one. When the ratio drops below three-to-one, the relationship is in trouble. I try applying this yardstick to my stressful relationship. I can't give it a passing grade. I am really tired of walking on eggshells around this person whose feathers are easily ruffled and who might give me a quick painful peck when I'm least expecting it.

Am I content with the chicken feed this relationship offers? What I really want is a more nourishing relationship, but it's time to nourish myself first.

Several of my women friends feel extremely stressed by their daughters-in-law, their mothers-in-law, their sisters-in-law. We choose our friends, but we don't choose our in-laws, and quite frankly, some of them are people we wouldn't choose at all. Still, we try to smile or get through the holiday dinners as best we can.

So I have a stressful relationship, and for my own

mental health, for my own bodily health, it is way past time for me to let go of this stressor. Just let it be what it is—close enough and distant enough—without wanting anything to be different and without wanting anything to change.

I get myself in trouble when I compare my relative to someone else's relative. Those other people have such a good relationship; I want that! Forgiveness is said to be giving up hope of having a different past, a different present, or a different future. I have to give up hope of having a different person.

This is one place where I lose faith in surrendering to Life. I don't want to give up on this person, I don't want to give up on this relationship, yet if I am going to give up my stress, it is time to simply let sleeping dogs lie. Let go. Let be. Surrender to Life, who has my long-term welfare at heart.

Finishing Unfinished Business

OOH, DO I even want to look into that dark box of Unfinished Business? It happened a while ago, maybe a long time ago. It's embarrassing. I feel ashamed. Maybe I'm still angry or resentful.

Nowadays, I try to stay current with my unfinished business. I aim to ask forgiveness quickly. But then there's that stuff that happened long ago.

Synchronistically, an old boyfriend, Harry, contacted me four months before my diagnosis. I used to think he was "the one." I used to think we were soul mates. Our parting, thirty years ago, was very hard for me, perhaps especially because he immediately went on to lead the life I had envisioned for "us."

Harry Facebooked me to ask if he could drop by for a visit while he was on the East Coast. I talked it over with Bill. I wondered to him whether Harry's marriage was on the rocks; Bill wondered to me whether Harry had received a diagnosis. Then I replied "Yes" to Harry.

He came by one afternoon when Bill wasn't home and stayed for three hours. We caught up on each other's lives. I asked his forgiveness; he asked mine.

Three weeks later, at a personal growth workshop, I received the assignment to write a letter, asking for forgiveness from someone, and to include a list of the gifts I had received from that person. I wrote my letter of amends to Harry and listed the good things that had come from him cutting me loose into the stream of my own life, even though I went kicking and screaming. (Literally. I feel very ashamed to think about it.) I sent him the letter. Two weeks later, I received it back, stamped *Paid In Full*. That guy always did have a sense of humor; that was one of things I loved about him.

Fortunately, that piece of unfinished business finished itself, but other little niches remain. Unfinished business includes wounds, resentments, hurts, and disappointments. It's way past time to forgive myself, ask the other person for forgiveness, and let the grievances all go, one by one.

Alcoholics Anonymous takes this matter of unfinished business very seriously. Step Eight states: Made a list of all persons we had harmed, and became willing to make amends to them all, and Step Nine says: Made direct amends to such people wherever possible, except when to do so would injure them or others.

The place to begin this atonement is by practicing self-forgiveness. "I forgive myself for not understanding . . ." is an easy and powerful practice. This was my main practice during a two-week retreat, and I found that it not only deepened my forgiveness, it also strengthened my self-compassion.

While the ego is strong, it thinks these little and big

owies of life don't matter that much. But emotional baggage is heavy. Now is the time to recognize it, forgive, and let go of that unfinished business.

You know how you feel when you finish a project. *Ahh. Done.* You can let it go and smile to yourself. When unfinished business is finished, you let it go, and it's gone. You walk on into life carrying less baggage and feeling lighter.

Surrendering to Life #3

WHEN I STARTED listing the gifts I had received from Harry, I began to look at my post-Harry life from a different angle. At the time, I could only see/feel that I had a big hole in my life. I compared my life to his. He got married; I was still single. In my late thirties, my dating life dried up to just about zero.

After my breakup with Harry, I left Portland, Oregon, where I had lived for three years, and I drove east to my home in Vermont, camping all the way. I followed, or tried to follow, the Nez Perce Trail, but signage was scarce-to-nonexistent and locals didn't know what I was talking about. *This trail needs a guidebook*, I thought to myself. One morning at a picnic table, I wrote down the budget that such an undertaking would require, but I couldn't figure out how I would ever have time in my life to write such a guidebook.

A year later, when my dad said, "You should write a book," and I said, "Well, I'd like to write a book on the Nez Perce trail," and he said, "Send me the budget," I did. Researching and writing that book was one of the purposes of my life. I feel strongly that it was one of the reasons why I was put on this earth. I could never have done it if I'd been coupled or had children. I could never have done it if I'd designed my own life and settled down in Portland with Harry. This is when I began to see that Life had a different plan for me than I had for myself. In my thirties, I thought I knew better than Life how to live it, but Life had a beautiful plan for me—one that totally resonated with my soul even more truly than my soul mate did.

As soon as I had finished my research travels, Life delivered Bill to me. Certainly, the Bill-package isn't the one I would have chosen off the shelf, but there he was and is, a loving companion on my life's journey, someone I immediately felt at home with.

Maybe I should just go ahead and surrender to Life, who seems to have truer and deeper answers to life's persistent little questions than I do.

Those Who Show Up

You've heard time and again, and perhaps you know from your own experience, that you're surprised by the people who show up in your time of need, and perhaps also disappointed by those who don't.

My sister sent me a big, gorgeous bouquet of flowers that lasted two weeks. The meditation center where I teach sent an orchid plant. But I was surprised by the student who left a tiny orchid on the front bench in the entry of our house. So sweet.

Neighbors brought over various versions of chicken soup, so I barely had to cook for the two weeks after my surgery.

Cards began to arrive in the mail. A card from Sandy, whom I worked with twenty-five years ago at a flower shop. Cards from cousins. A card from the garden club. Cards from writer friends. Cards from long-ago and faraway friends, and cards from neighbors who see me almost every day.

Some few of the cards missed the mark entirely, as the writers talked about fighting cancer, which I was not doing, but the message hardly mattered. Just to receive this prayer-on-a-notecard through the mail touched me deeply. I placed them all on my altar, where I could look at them and reread them every few days while I was on retreat.

Afterward, I'd see people in the parking lot or at the food co-op—perhaps we were only Facebook friends or Pilates acquaintances, but they would ask me how I was or say something personal about their own experience with cancer.

Eventually, I received a card from Harry, my ex-boyfriend, who had just reestablished contact after a thirty-year hiatus. "I sit in silence for you, my friend," he wrote.

Yes. That's really all there is to do now. Simply sit in silence and enjoy this one wild and precious life, full of friends, caring, love, and compassion.

Those Who Drop
Out of Sight

As for those friends and relatives I didn't hear from, I know very good and well that they were thinking about me. They can't hide from me, even though they were trying.

I'm sure some were stymied about what to say or what to write. How many sympathy and get-well cards have I myself not written, simply because I didn't know what to say or I was afraid I'd say the wrong thing. Doubt assails me. I want to be of comfort, but maybe I won't be.

I hesitate because I am unsure, and then my good intention falls off my radar screen. I procrastinate. I forget. I remember. I think, *Oh, it's too late.* The card that meant the most to me came two months "late." It goes to show that it's never too late. In fact, better late than never.

Of course, sometimes I practice the time-honored art of denial. I pretend I didn't hear, or I promptly forget. I don't want to "catch" their cancer, their illness, their trauma, and I certainly don't want to catch death, or maybe even *cause* someone's death. If I don't write, if I don't show up, if I don't say that one last thing to them, even if it's *I love you*, then as long as I haven't said it, maybe they won't die. (If I do say it, will I cause their death?) It is fascinating to consider how much magical thinking still dominates my actions.

Sometimes I content myself with "It's the thought that counts." A kind of mental Facebooking: *I heard. I know. I didn't click 'Like' because that seemed the wrong thing to click. Now what?* I am literally thinking of them, repeatedly.

Some people feel so ashamed of their own pain and loss that they cannot share themselves with others, and they feel they therefore cannot offer solace. Not writing a card is just another way for them to beat up on themselves. *Oh, they probably don't want a card from me, anyway.*

I compare myself to a friend who often manages to be in the inner circle of a sick or dying person; I'm always in the distant circle of acquaintances. *She's more important,* I think. *I'm not that important. She's a connector; I'm aloof.* Yet I felt so happy that distant acquaintances, people I barely knew, wrote to me.

In fact, all our friends and acquaintances are thinking of us, whether they want to or not. They are thinking of us whether they are open-hearted or closed-hearted. As human beings, our natural response is to feel the pain of others and put ourselves in their shoes, their perhaps very uncomfortable shoes, for at least a minute. The friends we don't hear from are the ones who need our compassion because they can't tolerate our pain, while we ourselves are at least bearing up. Their words, their note, their phone call would mean so much to us, yet they can't bring themselves to connect—with us or with their own pain.

Some of us can't tolerate feeling that pain, and we push away. Those of us who have been through the school of hard knocks don't believe our ego when it says *Wait!* or *Not yet* or *Later* or *I'm not sure*. Sometimes I sit down to write a line or two from my heartfelt mishmash, and I now see that this is the most precious gift I can give to someone who is suffering.

Power of Attorney

ONE OF THE things I wanted to get done was to change my power of attorney. My neighbor Connie is my durable power of attorney for health care, my sister is the trustee of my living trust (in hopes of avoiding probate), but what about those stray assets that would go to probate, that are simply in the name of "Cheryl Wilfong"?

I named Bill as my power of attorney three years ago, but recent events had confirmed my suspicions that Bill is a leaky vessel. He doesn't respond well to stress, and he's susceptible to scams. I needed, if not a tight-ass, at least someone who shared my Virgo (rising) enjoyment of details and would run a tight ship.

First of all, I wanted a new lawyer. Talk about letting go of stressful relationships! I knew it would take at least four months for my current lawyer to get around to doing the paperwork, and that would be after she finished tax season in mid-April, and then took a two-week vacation. Her office couldn't even find a record of the power of attorney that I signed there three years ago. No. I needed a relationship with someone who I felt cared about me.

In order to make an appointment with a new-to-me

estate lawyer whom several of my neighbors were using, I first had to take a two-hour workshop with him. Since the lawyer, who grew up in Putney (where Bill was a teaching colleague with his parents at The Putney School), has an office an hour away, this meant a four-hour chunk out of some day.

By the end of May, I signed the piece of paper appointing a new power of attorney. But then, my nominee was so overwhelmed by the twenty-three pages of boilerplate, plus my nine pages of instructions, that he bailed out.

My father hadn't wanted bankers, accountants, or lawyers charging their high fees to his estate, and I inherited the same prejudice. My Hoosier lawyer costs $375 an hour. Yes, she's worth it, but it's a lot of money.

Bill's little trust fund from his father grew not at all from the time of his father's death in 1971 until Bill received it at the time of his mother's death in 1995. Bill's mother's trust to him, which was originally set up with her local New Jersey bank, has gone through four bank mergers, with Bill's meager inheritance consistently being overlooked in favor of wealthier clients. Last year, it cost Bill $15,000 to break those trusts and get them transferred to our local Trust Company of Vermont. No, I wouldn't wish that scenario of "the professionals" on anyone.

It took another month before I found a friend willing to take on the POA responsibility. Then back to the estate lawyer, but this time I only required a fifteen-minute appointment.

My next mortality projects are to put my advance directives, including my durable power of attorney, on file online with the Vermont Registry, which feeds into a national registry. Two women from the *Being Mortal* book discussion group also want to update theirs, so maybe the three of us can get together this winter to support each other through this project.

Sitting down and actually doing these nonurgent projects requires strong intention. It's much more fun to do today's immortality projects of children and family or arts and crafts than to do the paperwork mortality projects for the coming day.

It's hard to imagine myself not having agency, not having control over my own life, yet this is what often happens. My father, who was always "the boss," lost his authority the month before he died. My mother slept during most of her last two months. Someone has to take the power when I have lost my own willpower, and that is the person I entrust with my power of attorney.

Racing with Nan

WHEN I WAS awaiting my turn for my second mammogram and dressed in a pink johnny, I saw Nan, also dressed in a johnny, coming out of the other dressing room. I hid my secret (*I'm here for my second mammogram*) behind normal chitchat. Nan and I are social acquaintances; we are friends of the same friends. So I wasn't surprised, three weeks later, to see Nan walk out of the Nurse Navigator's office just before I walked in. "Nan!" I exclaimed. In an instant, we each knew why the other one was there.

Kelly, the Nurse Navigator, rolled her eyes and shook her head. "We really try to prevent this from happening," she said, "but it's hard in a small town."

Nan had her lumpectomy the week before I had mine, but then somehow, she raced far ahead of me, so that by the time I was starting my seven weeks of radiation, she was finishing hers. I kept feeling that I was losing the time race. That was a stressful thought, followed by other subsidiary stressful thoughts.

Maybe Nan has a better chance of survival, because everything fell into place for her? Should I be worrying about micro-tumors growing in the two months between my surgery and the beginning of radiation?

Nurse Navigator Kelly assured me that as long as radiation happens within three months of the lumpectomy, survival rates are the same. I didn't need to worry about my slow dance toward radiation.

I worried that I might be losing the race for survival, but cancer was not running my life. *Life is not a race*, I had to keep reminding myself. My life was not being interrupted by cancer. I was living my life, and cancer was part of it. It was a problem child, to be sure. I just had to adjust my life around it. Life itself has a restorative, healing effect. My life included a retreat. The lives of other cancer patients included their child's wedding or a long-anticipated vacation. Life is part of our care plan, too. I was not on a deadline, though, of course, that is what the mind fears.

Each day we walk our walk, and quite frankly, everyone's destination is the same, no matter what name we call it or what detours we take. Let's enjoy the journey, the day-by-day walk, because, in one way or another, we are all headed for the finish line.

The Comparing Mind

A s FAR AS I can see, the comparing mind is the only mind we have, and it is usually extremely unhelpful, even stressful, too. Comparing myself to Nan and her quick treatment was useless. Comparing myself to Liz with her lower Oncotype DX score? Really useless. Her genes are her genes, and my genes are my genes.

I compare my experience to some imagined past. Useless. My past is my past. I compare my present to someone else's present. Also, really useless. I spend time imagining a lovely future for myself; or a horrible future for myself. Really, really useless.

When I wrote an essay about my financial legacy in writing group, irrepressible Lani said, "Hey, if you've got extra money, the Lani travel fund could use some." That's the comparing mind just doing its thing. It can't help it. *She has more money; I have less money.*

We compare how much money we have to how much someone else has. If they have more, we desire what they have. *Just think what I could do with that much money.* If they have less, we breathe a sigh of relief that we are not in their well-worn shoes.

For years now, I've practiced yoga with closed eyes.

If I look at other people, or even glance at them, my comparing mind will natter on. *Well, she's not very flexible* or *She's so much better than I am*. Comparing my body, my stretches, to anyone else's is also really useless. Closing my eyes quiets my mind and makes me more attentive to my own body.

Once in a while, while Bill and I are out for a walk or in some new place, he will say, "This reminds me of . . . ." When I compare this moment with a memory, I have lost the present moment. I am in the virtual reality of the mind, instead of the physical reality of the body. Perhaps you have been out for a walk in nature and heard someone say, "This reminds me of Disneyland." Yoo-hoo. Come back to the present moment, my friend. We want to savor the present moment, not compare it a memory.

As a writer, I use comparison all the time—it's called metaphor and simile. I depend on metaphor to summon up an image in the reader's mind. When I say that *comparing thoughts are attention thieves, they rob us of our lives*, you know they are not literal robbers, but suddenly you have an image in your mind, and due to the comparison, you understand something about how the mind uses comparison to understand experience, but also how the mind misuses comparison to distract itself and put people and places in unreal one-up/one-down, good/bad, black/white frames of reference. In truth, each thing, each person, each place *is*. Period.

I can't stop the comparing mind, since it's the only one I have. I can simply notice it. And when it tells me something—like "Nan got faster treatment" or "Liz got a lower score"—I don't have to believe it. I'm not less-than either one. I simply *am*—surrendering to Life as it is, one more time.

Surrendering to Life #4

WHEN I SAY I am surrendering to Life, I do not mean I am throwing in the towel. I do not mean I am waving the white flag of truce. I am not giving up. I am not giving in. I am not surrendering to cancer. I am surrendering to Life.

Life offers me some wonderful diagnostic tools, like the Oncotype DX test. Life offers me a smorgasbord of treatment options and drugs.

Of course I will do radiation. Radiation works. And sometimes it doesn't. Of course I will take a five-year drug. I might only take it for a few months or a few years. That remains to be seen. The side effects might be severe, or they might not. The drug usually works, and occasionally it doesn't.

Like the two chiropractors with metastasized cancers, I seek alternative treatments to complement the allopathic approach. I do things that make sense to me, although they might not make sense to other people.

I will go to the acupuncturist to treat the effects of radiation. I ask friends about naturopaths, even though naturopaths are not covered by Medicare. I will go to the alternative health care center, Cornucopia Choice, for services that are not available elsewhere, such as a test for the heavy metals in the body and the vitamin C infusions. I go to a masseuse every week as preventative maintenance. I live in a community that is rich with alternative practitioners.

Beyond these choices for treatments, I accept Life as it is unfolding. I submit to Life as if Life knows best, as if Life knows better than I do how to live it.

Acupuncture for Radiation

MY EDITOR, SUSAN, also a cancer survivor, recommended going to an acupuncturist every week as a preventative for the side effects of radiation. One of the reasons why I like to go to acupuncture is that Chinese medicine has its own view of the body. Janet, my acupuncturist, says puzzling things like "too much heat" or "not enough wind" in the body. When I went, she told me my liver and gall bladder pulses were tight. The liver has a pulse? Not characterized by a number—fast or slow—but by the word "tight." Hmmm.

I can understand, at least vaguely, the concept of the body having energy meridians that sometimes get clogged up. Occasionally, I discover a spot on my body that is exceedingly tender. I apply the pressure of my thumb—a sort of acupressure—in hopes of unclogging the energy traffic jam.

Janet said that studies show that cancers come and go in the body. An invasive cancer is invasive—it will kill you. But other cancers, including breast cancer, go into remission all on their own. We all have cancer cells floating around in our bodies. Sometimes our immune system takes care of them, and sometimes it doesn't. Sometimes cancers just hang out and don't do much of anything. A study of car-accident autopsies showed a surprising number of undiagnosed uterine and prostate cancers. We don't "get" cancer. We already have it. We just provoke it with irritants in our body from the environment.

Janet's point of view was that this whole vast breast-cancer business was a way to scare women into having surgery so that the medical establishment could make a lot of money. Hmmm. I'd never thought of it that way before.

Liz, a PhD who loves research and who is married to a physician, had just four weeks of a higher dose of radiation, six days a week, which is how it's done in Canada. Physicians in the United States generally prefer the seven-week course of radiation for breast cancer. Incidentally, the seven-week regimen earns a hospital $3,000 to $8,000 more per patient than the four-week course of treatment.

I asked Janet about vitamins and supplements. "Should I consider a special diet?" True to form, her answer bent my mind. "You don't have cancer now," she said. "You're here to support your body through the radiation treatment. Radiation is the issue."

Well, uh, yes.

Janet offered me some "radio support" supplements—the first supplements she's sold me in the fifteen years I've been seeing her. I usually visit her a couple of times a year for some random symptom or other that would make no sense to a medical doctor.

I lay down on her table and relaxed. I felt the bee sting of the needles as she placed them in my ankles and wrists. Then she left the room, and I gazed out the window to the blue sky and Mount Wantastiquet on the other side of the Connecticut river. I dozed off for twenty minutes.

Yes, I felt I was in good hands.

Radiation with Evelyn

O<small>N</small> A<small>PRIL</small> 6, I went to the oncologist, who made an appointment for me to see the radiologist three weeks later. Three weeks! Everything had gone so smoothly and efficiently, and now I had to wait for three weeks to take the next step. I called the radiology office for an earlier appointment. "We'll put you on our call list, in case anyone cancels." The next week, while I was in Keene, I dropped by the radiology department, hoping personal contact might speed things up. "Oh, yes, we have your name on our call list." I never did get called.

Meanwhile, I went out to lunch with Evelyn, who, at age seventy-nine, was having her fourth go-round with lymphoma. She was starting radiation just a few days before me. In between bites of her chicken sandwich (she was trying to put on weight), she said, "I hope I have another year or two." She said it with such perfect equanimity, as befits a long-term meditator, that my heart melted. I didn't feel sad; I simply felt the preciousness of the moment. *Oh, right*, I thought. *Evelyn might not have much time left.*

"Let's see if we can get back-to-back appointments for radiation," I said.

I knew that people in cancer support groups live longer than people who don't belong to support groups. The local hospitals offer these support groups; and my good friend Fritze had spent six years in the one in Keene offering hope to newly-diagnosed cancer patients.

Somehow, though, a support group didn't particularly appeal to me. For one thing, my schedule was already quite full, and spending two hours every weekday going to and from radiation was putting many other projects on hold. But the idea of having my support group with Evelyn every day during our forty-minute drive to Keene, and forty minutes back to Brattleboro, seemed just right. We could talk Dharma, *dukkha* (stress), radiation side effects, and life.

Eight weeks after my lumpectomy, I finally got in to see the radiologist. The head radiation technician, Erica, took me into a machine, lined me up, and tattooed my torso with three blue dots so that the lasers would line me up in the exact same position every time. One blue dot on each side of my rib cage to make sure I was lying flat, and one blue dot on my right breast to make sure I was aligned vertically as well as horizontally. With the target of my torso perfectly positioned, radiation could aim precisely at the site of my surgery.

I have tattoos, I crowed on Facebook. Well, just barely. They looked like tiny blue freckles.

Then another week passed before my treatments could begin. "Can you speed that up?" I asked.

"No. Lots of people have to sign off."

Oh. I could imagine the behind-the-scenes approval processes that needed to happen.

I waited one more week, and finally, finally, I went to my first radiation appointment. "Can I get an appointment near Evelyn?" I asked.

The radiation technicians waffled. "Evelyn who?" and "Well, if Evelyn asks us, we might be able to."

Oh, right. What if I were an overbearing person who wanted to carpool with Evelyn, but she didn't want to carpool with me?

I called Evelyn. "You have to ask them for back-to-back appointments," I said. She said she would.

Two days later, we were set. Our appointments weren't quite back-to-back—there was one person in between us—but it was close enough that we could carpool, and Evelyn would then wait the extra twenty minutes for me.

"I want to drive," said Evelyn, "because I may not feel like driving later. And I have gas cards from the Nurse Navigator at the hospital." I nodded. Evelyn's been through her chemotherapy and radiation process three times before. She knew how things worked. As it turned out, she drove almost every day.

The radiation table was a hard-plastic bed, covered in a hospital sheet. As I lay on my back, the four radiation technicians placed a triangular bolster under my knees. I draped my arms on arm stirrups above me where they would be out of the way. Then I was looking up at the ceiling with its large translucent picture of a spring garden—daffodils, tulips, grape hyacinths, all in full bloom, with crab apple and cherry blossoms above, and a pond in the middle.

After the technicians adjusted me, and double-checked with each other to make sure I was lined up, and that the radiation apparatus was precisely 97.6 centimeters above my breast, I lay there with a bare right breast, looking up at the ceiling garden. When I heard the heavy door close, and I was left alone in the room, I could feel my body relax one more notch.

As the radiating apparatus automatically moved into position for its thirty-seven-second scan, the words of a loving-kindness chant came to mind: "Radiating kindness over the entire world." I focused on one of the daffodil trumpets and imagined it radiating golden light and kindness as I sang to myself in my mind, "Radiating kindness over the entire world." The radiation was still buzzing as it arced from left to right over my chest, finishing with several seconds aimed at the scar on the right side of my right breast, so I continued with the next lines of the chant: "Radiating kindness over the entire world, spreading upwards to the skies and downwards to the depths. Outwards and unbounded, freed from hatred and ill-will."

I imagined the radiation beam pervading my breast, and I could actually feel the sound of the light buzz throughout my body. Then I imagined the radiation spreading throughout the room. Why else did the radiation technicians leave the room? I imagined kindness radiating beyond the room, out to the four very kind technicians, and to the waiting room where Evelyn sat waiting for me. Radiating out to the reception area, where the receptionists already knew me by sight. Radiating kindness out to the Ashuelot River behind the hospital, and over the entire world.

Then the buzzing was over. The technicians came in to lower the bed. I got up, went to the dressing room, put my johnny into the dirty-clothes hamper, and got dressed.

Then I was standing beside Evelyn in the waiting room. "Okay. I'm ready."

No matter how this story turns out, I'm ready.

Evelyn's Last Day of Radiation

AFTER EVELYN'S FINAL radiation treatment in Keene, I took her out to brunch. We went to Timoleon's, a restaurant that has one long counter, seven booths, and a handful of tables beside the front window that faces Main Street. At 10:30, the place was nearly full.

We were shown to our table by the proprietor, who seemed sprightly despite his bent spine and his trousers hiked up to the bottom of his ribcage. Our waitress had long black hair, was thin as a cigarette, and couldn't have been a day under eighty. She reminded me of Morticia Addams. She knew almost everyone in the booths as she walked around pouring coffee. I appeared to be almost the youngest person there, even at age sixty-seven. While Evelyn and I were waiting for our chipped beef on toast (me) and Belgian waffles (Evelyn), a woman with a little oxygen tank pushed her walker ahead of her to a nearby booth.

"Boy, did we come to the right place!" I said to Evelyn. "There are Heavenly Messengers everywhere."

We looked around us at the various varieties of aging.

The place was buzzing. A bald man was just standing up from his booth; he had to pause for a minute to straighten up and let his joints lubricate themselves before he could start walking. I looked at a nearby thirty-something man for a while before I realized he had a white cane with a red tip, and the woman he was sitting with was probably his case manager.

I glanced down at the paper place mat with two dozen ads for local services—more Heavenly Messengers! Aging was represented by lawn care services—I assumed for those no longer able to do their outdoor chores themselves—and also by the financial advisor "Serving the Investment Needs of the Community." Illness was represented by the ad for a local insurance agent—"Don't Buy Your Medicare Supplement Until You Talk To Me!" Death was represented by Keene Monument Co., Custom Marble & Granite. "We Make Memories Last."

Evelyn and I smiled at each other. We, too, were walking Heavenly Messengers.

Ride to Radiation

EVELYN REQUIRED ONLY five weeks of radiation, and she got started a week before I did, so after a month of car-pooling, I was on my own for the next three weeks. Over the previous couple of months several women had offered to drive me to radiation, but I didn't feel that I needed their help. I was feeling pretty good; the expected fatigue had not yet set in. *Oh, I'll drive myself,* I thought. A forty-minute commute to a fifteen-minute appointment is easy.

On Tuesday of my first solo week, I hiked the mile into Pisgah State Park to go swimming in Kilburn Pond with my neighbor Connie. Her brother Jimmy and sister-in-law Laura met us there.

"Oh, Laura," I said. "You have a high-top bathing suit! I need one of those. Where did you get it?"

Laura was wearing a navy-blue Speedo-type swimsuit, which completely covered her breasts. Since sunlight can "recall" the radiation, even years after radiation, I now needed to cover up my radiated breast. This meant no more flaunting of my cleavage, at least in the broad daylight of a hot sun, for the rest of my life.

While Laura, Connie, and I were companionably

swimming over to the granite outcroppings on the other side, Laura told me, "I want to drive you to your radiation appointments on Thursday and Friday." Laura had had ovarian cancer three years earlier with a follow-up of chemotherapy. During her treatment, she didn't allow friends into her house because of her weakened immune system, but she did go walking every day that winter with a different friend.

"Oh, that's okay," I said. "I can drive myself."

"No," said mild-mannered Laura. "I want to drive you on Thursday and Friday. What time is your appointment?"

That's when it dawned on me that receiving a ride was not a failure of my self-sufficiency. When I arrived home later that afternoon, I posted on Facebook, "Do you want to drive me to radiation in Keene?" In less than two days, my dance card was full, and people were still messaging me that they wanted to give me a ride to radiation. When Bill heard about so many other people driving me, he also wanted to take me one day.

The women who responded surprised me. Marilyn, who attended a reiki workshop with me twelve years ago, was a former nurse. Gloria, who was in my writing group fifteen years ago and whom I occasionally see at a play, offered to drive one day. Come to find out, her daughter had cancer while Gloria lived in Maine. So, in a way, Gloria was expressing her gratitude to all her daughter's friends who took her to her appointments while Gloria lived six hours away.

In addition to local women, I received messages from

my far-flung relatives. Leslie in Tennessee said, "I wish I lived closer." Carol Jean, who had breast cancer seventeen years ago in northern Indiana, wrote, "I'd be glad to take you if I could." My cousin Susan in Colorado said, "I'd drive you if I lived closer." My heart was warmed by these messages of caring. Receiving a ride to radiation—real or virtual—made me feel cared for by a community of friends and family that extended far and wide.

Fatigue

SEVERAL WOMEN TOLD me about the fatigue that accompanies radiation and sets in after about four weeks of treatment. One friend said she needed about a month after the end of her radiation treatments to recover, to just kick back, rest, read books, and go nowhere.

Hmmm. Going nowhere did not sound like my summer schedule.

Susan, the editor of *The Meditative Gardener*, told me she had chemotherapy followed by radiation, but that she had acupuncture along with radiation and did not feel fatigued. So I went for weekly acupuncture.

I was scheduled to go on a four-day retreat two days after the end of radiation, and the retreat manager kindly waited for me to make my final decision, but she needed to know, for certain, two weeks before the retreat began. Well, if I wanted a cheaper flight to Virginia, I'd have to decide two weeks in advance anyway.

Halfway through radiation, I was taking a half-hour nap on the sofa every afternoon. Nothing new there. Then I began to sag after every meal so I'd take a twenty-minute nap mid-morning, another twenty-minute nap mid-afternoon, and a thirty-minute nap after dinner. I love naps. Even a ten-minute nap pushes the reset button. Beforehand, I am dragging, and afterward I'm awake, I'm alert and refreshed. Three naps a day felt like three desserts a day. On many days, I went out to the hammock beside the vegetable garden, covered myself with a light sheet, and dozed off to the sound of birds singing in the trees.

Was this it? Was this the fatigue they talked about?

I made my plane reservation for Virginia. I can nap on an airplane. I usually drift off while the plane is taxiing for takeoff, and I wake up when the drinks are being served.

As soon as I was through with radiation, I returned to my usual routine of just one nap every afternoon.

One possible explanation for my lack of fatigue is that the naturopath put me on 20 mg of Melatonin every night. That's ten times the usual dose I take for jet lag. Melatonin has been shown to have an anti-cancer effect. Maybe I was sleeping really well every night?

Or here's another theory. I continued with my three circus classes every week, plus a Pilates class, plus a yoga class, and I added in a clown class, because laughter is supposed to be the best medicine. Maybe a strong dose of endorphins five days a week helped keep fatigue at bay?

One evening, during trapeze class, I was so weary from nearly three hours of exercise that I took a thirty-second nap on the mat in between tricks. That is the shortest power nap I have ever taken, but it immediately revived me.

My psychoanalyst friend Liz, who teaches meditation, says that anxiety contributes to fatigue. Holding tension in the body from each and every stressful thought is exhausting. Less stress leads to less fatigue.

Every day on the radiation bed I was super-relaxed, pervading myself and the world with loving-kindness. I have no doubt that my meditation practice supported my mind as well as my body. I kept my mind close to the present moment. There was no worry, no fear, no anxiety to speak of. While my mind was going nowhere, my body could relax.

Whatever the reason for having so little fatigue, I feel extremely grateful to my body, my meditative mind, and my team of health-care, alternative-care, and circus-care professionals.

The End of Radiation

FRIDAY, JUNE 19, was my thirty-third and last day of radiation treatment. The day before, I had been in the hospice thrift store, Experienced Goods, looking for capri pants, and there they were—pale, pale pink silk, sprinkled with a pattern of fuchsia and pale-yellow flowers with turquoise leaves. The pants fit, so I bought them for four dollars. I dubbed them my party pants for their bright cheeriness. Wearing them on my last day of radiation made me feel dressed up and happy to boot.

Evelyn took me out for breakfast. The radiation technicians presented me with a Certificate of Completion. I gave them each a copy of my book, *The Meditative Gardener*. We hugged. My women's group had lunch at an outdoor cafe, and we gabbed for three hours. Bill took me out for dinner at The Marina restaurant on the West River, and then we went to a play.

No longer do I have to drive forty minutes to the hospital in Keene every weekday. No longer do I zip in and out of the caring hands of four radiation technicians for five minutes every day. Cancer has been removed from my breast. The beautiful scar on the right side of my right breast is now a red lightning bolt, and the puckery lymph node scar three inches away in my underarm is swollen red and hot.

If I held a Geiger counter to my right breast, would it click and hiss? What's the half-life of radiation treatments? They say the radiation is cumulative—I had thirty-three treatments, each one lasting thirty-seven seconds—so that they intensify, and the burn keeps on burning even after I receive my certificate of completion. Evelyn says she cannot get a PET scan to gauge the size of her lymphoma tumors until three months post-radiation. Any earlier, and the PET scan would throw off false positives. How long do electrons and neutrons still bounce around inside my right breast? The surgeon says that the effects of radiation can last as long as three years.

Even though Friday was a day of four graduation parties, I didn't really feel the celebration until the following Monday. A Monday where I did not have to drive to the hospital. A free Monday. A freed Monday. Ahhh. Radiation was really over. Now I could have my life back. Now I could go back to living.

The first day of summer arrived, and I have been warned not to expose my right breast to the sun lest I get "radiation recall"—the sun's rays retriggering the radiation and its side effects. My aerialist friend Crystal, age forty-two, who had cancer when she was sixteen, tells me her skin gets all funny if she exposes it to the sun.

My surgery has been done. The acupuncturist tells me she's not treating me for breast cancer, because I no longer have it. That's a refreshing point of view. She's treating me for radiation, and, in fact, the radiation fatigue that so many women report hasn't struck me.

I no longer have cancer—it has been removed: clear margins and clear lymph nodes. I'm no longer in radiation. Soon the oncologist will give me a prescription for the drug I will take for the next five years—I don't know for sure which one. I don't need to know. The oncologist hasn't given it or me a second thought. I have to trust her educated guess. She's been doing this for decades.

For now, all I need to know is that I've graduated. I can see the end of this conveyor belt that I've been on for the past five months. I am returning to ordinary life, where I am no longer a diagnosis, where I am no longer a problem to be solved. I can recommence *living* my life—a life all the more worth living each and every day, because I have seen that my renewed lease on life will indeed expire. Not yet. Perhaps not soon. But soon enough, of its own accord, the body will reach its expiration date.

As I face the land of the unknown future, I feel as if I were just learning to walk again. I've been held by the caring hands of so many medical professionals in the past few months, guiding my every step, and I feel deep affection for every one of them. Now I'm on my own. There's nothing more to *do* for the time being. In a way, I can't believe I'm "done." I'm really safe in my body now? I was on red alert, but now I have the green light to go by myself, out into the oh-so-green summer.

Can I keep my eyes on the journey and not on the goal of living to a ripe old age? Can I realize that with each moment, as Thich Nhat Hanh says, "I have arrived. I am home." I am safe at home in this very body.

Home sweet home. Body sweet body.

*Life is no longer a problem to be solved,
but a reality to be experienced.*

— SÖREN KIRKEGAARD

Going Public
on the Trapeze

I N MID-MAY, I received an e-mail from Wendy, who is on the board of the New England Center for Circus Arts. NECCA was having a fund-raiser the following week. Would I do a trapeze performance?

"Sure," I replied. This meant that I needed to set up three private lessons to figure out my routine and pressure Bill, who is a concert pianist, to play some nice slow piano music. We eventually used my iPhone to record him playing a section of a Debussy suite for piano.

Just two weeks earlier, the week that I started radiation treatment, I had begun taking a clown class with Nettie Lane on Monday evenings, figuring I could use all the endorphins I could get. An hour and a half of silliness every Monday would surely provide that. Four weeks later, on the day before my trapeze performance, Nettie coached my private lesson. She encouraged me to add a script to my routine, and together we came up with ten lines. The first was given while I was hanging upside down by one knee on the trapeze bar: "Hello. My name is Cheryl."

After seven days of daily practice, I had a rope burn on my back from one of my tricks, and another bar burn under my left knee, which held all my weight as I suddenly turned upside-down for the final trick in my act. In addition to being bruised, my body was cooked by the Radarange of radiation, so I had to practice my script while imagining my routine in my mind. On the day of my performance, I spent my entire thirty-five-minute commute to the jail where I teach meditation on Thursday afternoon, and the thirty-five minutes back as well, running through my script out loud and my routine in my mind—over and over again.

I arrived at the gymnasium in time to rehearse my routine once through. I had not had time to memorize Bill's Debussy accompaniment and to know which trick synced with which phrase of music, so I just had to hope for the best.

The fund-raiser began at 5:30. A twelve-year-old girl performed on the rope. A fifteen-year-old boy performed flawlessly on the handstand blocks. I was old enough to be their grandmother. Then it was my turn. Hey, it was a fund-raiser.

Everyone in the audience was over sixty. I knew about half of them. They laughed at my line that "circus has lowered my cholesterol," and they chuckled when I said that "circus is a fun way of building strong bones." All those menopausal women in the audience already had osteopenia, I was pretty sure. But the moment I really got to them was when I held my body vertically in front of the trapeze—one arm straight, hand gripping the bar; the other arm outstretched (behind the rope) as if flying; breasts and heart pointed straight toward the audience—and said that I had recently had surgery for breast cancer. Just before my final trick, I said that I was halfway through my radiation treatments. For this, they gave me a standing ovation.[*]

This script fit the mission of the circus school beautifully. Though the New England Center for Circus Arts is known for training professionals who go on to perform with the likes of Cirque du Soleil and for training teachers of the aerial arts, they do have several community programs, such as one for high school students and one for cancer survivors. My essential message was: *Hey, you retired people! You can do this too! It's good for you!* Circus is a really fun way to feel your endorphins, those natural opioids within the body that reduce stress and pain.

Of course, the intense focus on my performance for a week meant that even more loose ends were collecting. So many things left undone—writing projects, gardening projects, committee meetings that conflicted with my radiation appointments. But who was counting those? I was flying high with all those exercise endorphins and happy to be of service to an organization I love.

---

[*] You can see my performance on YouTube. Search for "Cheryl Wilfong."

Daily Life

I WAS PRETTY WELL able to live my ordinary life until radiation started at the beginning of May, and this time felt like a gift, a sort of vacation, a stay-cation at home.

My ordinary life is fairly busy on Tuesdays, Wednesdays, and Thursdays with a routine of my own choosing. On Monday, I go to Pilates. On Friday, I stay home if I can.

Usually, I arise before the sun and meditate for forty minutes. At 7:00 A.M., I turn on the computer and write my blog. At 8:00, I walk a quarter-mile to my neighbor's house, where three or eight of us gather to chitchat and then meditate for twenty minutes. If possible, I like to stay home in the morning to work on writing projects or other paperwork.

On Tuesday afternoons, I go to a meditation and writing group in Keene, New Hampshire, half an hour away. Afterward, I teach meditation at the county jail, on the women's block. Then I either teach a meditation class or go to yoga.

Wednesdays begin with a three-hour writing group. On Wednesday evenings I take two classes at the circus school—Circus Fitness and Trapeze 101. On Thursdays, I have my weekly massage and one more circus class—Flexibility 101.

Two Sundays a month, I give a Dharma talk, and I spend the preceding Saturday writing it.

Some various committees meet every couple of months; I volunteer for hospice occasionally; and, as a Master Gardener, I give gardening talks somewhere in the community every few months. In the winter, I volunteer for the emergency shelter at the Baptist church on Monday nights from one in the morning until closing time at 7:00 A.M.

This is the rough outline of how I spend the precious time of my ordinary life.

Now as to my list of projects:

In February, I finished the manuscript for *The Real Dirt on Composting* and sent it off to the editor. This was a collection of sixty-five essays on the art, science, and patience of composting. At the end of the month, I sent the edited manuscript to my favorite proofreader, and then to the book designer. Meanwhile, I sent my edited manuscript for a 365-day inspirational book, *Garden Wisdom 365 Days*, to several meditation teachers for endorsements. Then I sent the PDF of the manuscript, plus a book proposal, to two publishers.

While I was waiting for the manuscript of *Garden Wisdom* to work through its channels, I began researching another book I'd like to write, about going on retreat.

In March, two days after surgery, I began my

retreat—two weeks of self-retreat at home, followed by one week at Insight Meditation Society, followed by one weekend of teaching at Southern Dharma Retreat Center near Hot Springs, North Carolina, followed by five days of self-retreat at home, and ending with a week-long retreat at the Barre Center for Buddhist Studies. Bill loved the fact that I was having so much of my retreat in our guest suite, thirty feet away from the house. During what would normally be my walking meditation periods, I was stoking the wood stove, shoveling the walks, and hammering the ice dams off the roof.

The last of the snow finally melted during the first week of April, and mud season ended, in time for gardening season to begin the second week of April. Thank goodness for Elisha, the gardener who keeps my gardens in shape. The local garden club, Perennial Swappers, comes to tour my gardens on the first Thursday in May. It's always a race to get the flowerbeds ready for company.

While Elisha was mulching the flowerbeds, I worked on TurboTax. It takes me about a week of shuffling my Quicken numbers around to do my taxes, but, as a former accountant, I actually like to prepare my own tax return.

The third week of April, *The Real Dirt on Composting* came back from the designer. After a few tweaks, she uploaded it to the publisher. When two boxes of a hundred books arrived, I sent off to the Garden Writers Association for mailing labels addressed to garden writers who write columns in their local newspapers. Then I had second thoughts. This was the beginning of the loose ends. What I really should do, I thought, is pay $180 to send an e-mail announcement to all garden writers and offer them the opportunity to either download a free copy to their Kindle or e-mail me for a free hard copy, but I wasn't sure how to use Dropbox for the free download. That project went straight to the sidelines.

Radiation began on May 4, and that meant that every day had a two-hour bite out of it—fifty minutes to travel to a radiation appointment that lasted for twenty minutes, and fifty minutes back. This is when things to do really began to pile up.

I was the registrar for a retreat of my Community Dharma Leader peers from May 15 to 20. Fortunately, it was just an hour away, so I commuted to radiation every morning and was still on retreat for the remaining twenty-one hours of each day.

A week later, I did a solo trapeze performance at a fund-raiser for the New England Center for Circus Arts.

The day after my trapeze performance, despite Bill's skepticism I bought a new car—actually a used electric car, a three-year-old Nissan Leaf with 7,600 miles—for $13,000. The price sounded too good to be true. Was it a lemon? This meant ordering an electric charger online, and then waiting for the electrician to come install a 220-volt outlet in the garage. Another project waiting on the sidelines.

I soon received a letter from the insurance company: "You have more cars than drivers. Please explain." I was waiting for Bill's decision as to whether to sell his fourteen-year-old Prius or my eleven-year-old Prius, which had more miles on it. Another project went to the sidelines.

My neighbor Orly invited me to present a workshop at the Slow Living Summit in early June, which precedes Brattleboro's Strolling of the Heifers parade and weekend of celebrating local agriculture. I proposed a workshop on Slow Composting, but instead was put on a panel with an herbalist and a locavore gardener. I tried to figure out how to weave mindfulness into that discussion. Finally, I volunteered to be the moderator for the panel.

At the beginning of June, I asked the volunteer administrator of the meditation center to change the date of the day-long retreat I was supposed to teach on June 21 to a week later. I wasn't sure that I would have the energy to teach just two days after ending radiation. They say that the fatigue as well as radiation burn sets in during the last two weeks.

The administrator agreed, but then nothing happened. I asked again the following week, and still received no answer. That's when I realized I would indeed be teaching on June 21 and then flying that evening to Virginia to attend one last four-day retreat with a meditation teacher I had been studying with for the past eight years, because he was retiring.

I had a choice between two responses in this situation: *Oh, no!* and *Oh. Hmmm. Yes.*

Oh, no! resists the way Life is unfolding. *Oh, no!* is straight-out stressful.

Oh. Hmmm. Yes. commits to any available happiness, of which I was having a surplus: End of radiation. *Yes!* No fatigue. *Yes!* Teaching a day-long writing retreat. *Yes!* Going on retreat. *Yes!*

I must admit, Life did a pretty good job of living me in my daily life during radiation, despite all my unraveled loose ends.

List of My Loose Ends

- gardening—dividing plants in the flower beds and taking the extras to plant sales at the library and at the garden club. Usually I give away four truckloads; this year I managed only one.
- painting touch-ups—the painter won't be available until July.
- gardening—flowers (from the compost) are growing in the vegetable garden. Either I need to transplant the flowers to the flowerbeds or convert the vegetable garden to a flower garden.
- insulating the attic—last winter was extra cold and a plastic hot-water pipe froze.
- electric outlets—but before insulation can proceed, a few more electrical outlets need to be installed.
- planting grass seed (I'm lobbying for clover) after a section of new stone wall has been built.
- yoga—I stopped going to yoga with Bill on Wednesday evenings because my trapeze class changed to Wednesday evening.
- voles devouring my broccoli, cabbage, and kale seedlings. I either need to ask Bill to trap the voles,

do it myself, get a new fence, install an electric fence, or throw my hands up in the air.

- Bill's rash remained an unfinished project—I force-fed him an alkaline diet (the Dr. Rau diet) for a week. I made an appointment for him with the acupuncturist. He went twice. I begged him to go to a fancier specialist at Dartmouth-Hitchcock. He canceled that appointment.

- I had to cancel a Master Gardener talk I was going to give about my new book, *The Real Dirt on Composting*, because it conflicted with my radiation appointment.

- book project—I abandoned my search for publishers for my manuscript *Garden Wisdom 365 Days*, an inspirational day-by-day book about mindfulness in the garden. This project is at the bottom of my to-do pile.

- electricity credits—Because we have fifty-nine solar photovoltaic panels on our roof, we have a $1,500 credit balance with the electric company, and we cannot get the money in cash. Bill kept nagging me to form a group with one of our neighbors, so that my credit balance could pay their electric bill, and they in turn could pay me. Ugh. Paperwork and a bunch of phone calls. I called the solar installer, and the receptionist said, "Buy an electric car."

I love all these things—my garden, my home, my health, Bill, writing—yet I simply couldn't juggle everything. So I let Life make my decisions for me. Some things happened, and some did not. Sometimes Life picked up the phone to make a call; sometimes she didn't. Sometimes Life went out to the garden; sometimes she didn't. Various sheets of paper piled up on my desk in the kitchen. Sometimes Life would pick one up, but often she simply forgot what was in the pile.

I surrendered my list of Things To Do; I surrendered my idea of loose ends; I surrendered my idea of being the doer who does things. I simply watched as some things got done, and other ideas of things-to-do continued to rattle around in my mind.

Bill's To-Do List

NEEDLESS TO SAY, my relaxed, surrendering-to-Life approach did not always fit well with the person I play house with. He wanted me to do what needs to be done, and he wanted it done now or in the very near future. He still thinks there is a doer. He thinks, reasonably, that *I* am that doer. I used to think so, too.

"So when are you going to . . . ?" he would ask.

"I can't do it this morning," I replied. "I have to go to radiation."

He narrowed his eyes. "So when *are* you going to do it?"

"I don't know." I say this because I want to be honest. I really don't know.

"Just tell me when."

The conversation might go downhill from there, or maybe he'll stalk off, grumbling.

Our relationship is one of parallel play. I dig in the gardens; he prunes and cuts down the trees in the background. I cook; he plays his piano. He washes dishes; I go to my computer keyboard. But in the realm of house and yard maintenance, I was not keeping up my end of the bargain.

I was following my will-o-the-wisp instead of my will, and so I was responding in a very hit-or-miss fashion. I would start a project but leave it half finished. Mostly, chores kept drifting along in their incompleteness.

"Do it! Just do it!" he would order me. "*Please,*" he whined.

"I can't promise you," I replied.

His priority list was obviously different from my lack of priorities.

"When can you do it?" he would plead.

"I just don't know. Look at my calendar."

"On the iPad? You know I don't know how to find it. Here. You look at it." He thrust the iPad in my direction.

I sighed.

He sighed.

We nonverbally agree to pause this conversation, which is going nowhere. We stop at the crossroads before cross words are spoken. Neither of us wants to take either the fork in the road toward an ultimatum, or the fork in the road toward giving in or giving up. We pause.

To be continued some other day.

Vitamin C Infusions

S EVERAL OF MY friends who have had cancer have gone to the local Cornucopia Choice Holistic Health Center for vitamin C infusions, so I decided to go there, too. I now receive a weekly dose of 40,000 mg of vitamin C by IV, straight into the veins. Within five seconds, vitamin C is in the tide of my bloodstream, washing over my entire body.

If you tried to take that much vitamin C by mouth, it would give you diarrhea. Only about a third of the vitamin C we ingest makes it past the liver, which is busy cleaning vitamin C out of the bloodstream. This is the reason it's said that vitamin C only lasts for an hour in the body. The infused vitamin C continues to circulate for six to eight hours.

The megadose of vitamin C combines with the natural copper and iron of the body to form hydrogen peroxide, H_2O_2. Healthy cells can defend themselves from the resulting bath of hydrogen peroxide by calling on an enzyme called catalase. But cancer cells cannot defend themselves, and they die at the touch of hydrogen peroxide. It sounds like an inner antiseptic, which is probably why my energy sinks as soon as the needle goes into my vein.

I like the idea of vitamin C, and my oncologist simply nodded her head when I told her I was doing these infusions. I remember Linus Pauling, winner of a Nobel Prize for chemistry and a Nobel Peace Prize, promoting megadoses of vitamin C in the 1960s and '70s. Although the clinical trials for vitamin C efficacy remain sketchy, the American Cancer Society considers it an adjuvant (auxiliary) treatment.

Vitamin C is an antioxidant; we could say it prevents the body from rusting. One friend who is taking 8,000 mg a day for her Lyme disease says the brown spots on her skin are fading. But these vitamin C infusions are pro-oxidant rather than antioxidant, and for an hour or so, they are oxidizing my body from the inside. I think it's worth the price.

Evelyn and I are on the road again, once a week, this time to the Cornucopia Choice Holistic Health Center. Once again, we have back-to-back appointments, this time in neighboring recliners. We are still talking Dharma and *dukkha* and comparing notes on life.

Vitamin C for the Big C. Why not?*

---

* For more information about vitamin C infusions, go to the University of Kansas School of Medicine website: http://www.kumc.edu/school-of-medicine/integrative-medicine/patient-services/infusion-clinic.html.

Heavy Metals

THE NURSE AT the Cornucopia Choice Holistic Health Center wanted me to do a urine test for heavy metals. It so happened I had already done one, fifteen years earlier, when I was deciding whether or not to get a root canal. Back then, I was also deciding whether to go to Mexico to get all my fillings replaced, but my results were all in the normal range. Now, the nurse was particularly interested in comparing the results of the two tests.

When the findings came back this time, I was surprised to learn that I had four times the normal amount of lead in my system. I was also above average in thallium, which I had never even heard of.

Since the Industrial Age began, all sorts of heavy metals have been let loose in our environment, which means we all are carrying around more arsenic, zinc, and mercury in our bodies than our ancestors did. It's called "body burden." In 2004, Bill's daughter Jenifer McKim wrote an award-winning story on lead in candy from Mexico.* It turned out that the hot peppers used in making the candy were grown in lead-contaminated soil.

---

* Jenifer is an investigative reporter, and her story was a runner-up for the Pulitzer Prize in 2005.

Many of these heavy metals are endocrine disrupters. Lead (and zinc, too) mimics estrogen and can replace estrogen in the body, particularly in the bones. Research does not clearly conclude that lead is a carcinogen, but I have my suspicions.

You've probably heard the story about the ninety-eight-year-old woman who is diagnosed with breast cancer and then cries, "Why me?"

The "why" question is not particularly helpful, but of course that's where my mind goes. The answer that "I am of the nature to have disease" barely makes a dent in the mind's wanting to know, wanting to know for sure, wanting a scientific explanation. This is what the mind does: it seeks answers. And sometimes we are satisfied with half-baked answers. Too much lead in the body disrupting the endocrine system is a story that has a certain logic, a certain coherence, and so, although I wouldn't stake my life on it (even though maybe I should), I accept this answer of "too much lead" as the (unproven) carcinogen in my body.

Where the lead in my body comes from remains a mystery to me. My house is new enough (1979) that it was painted after lead paint was outlawed in 1978. Leaded gasoline is a thing of the past (as of 1986). Lead pipes and lead soldering may still be in use in city pipes, but out here in the country my water pipes are copper or PVC.

So how to get the lead out? The naturopath has given me several supplements to help with chelation, a process that uses particular ions to bind with the offending metal and thereby render it inert so that it can be passed out of the body without further damage. I sprinkle citrus pectin on my cereal and take several green chlorella tablets every day. In addition, I need to take a clay bath once a week to draw out the toxins, and I can also sweat out the toxic metals by using a far-infrared sauna.

Those are the remedies for my personal lead-abatement program to try to unburden my body of a heavy metal and lead it into health.

Rat Poison

T HALLIUM IS A rat poison, and, for some unknown reason, I have too much of it floating around in my body.

I am reminded of what Pema Chödrön says: "Holding a grudge is like eating rat poison and expecting the rat to die." I confess that for way too long, I've been holding a grudge against the most difficult and stressful person in my life. And now I have this very tangible reminder of how I am poisoning my mind (and thereby my body?) with irritation, frustration, and impatience. *STOP it, Cheryl! Just drop it. Let it be.*

First, let me remind myself that guilt about being a "bad" person, the kind who holds a grudge, is utterly useless here. Being averse to the aversive mind-states of anger only deepens the rut of aversion. I'm trying to extract myself from aversion, not dig a deeper hole.

I simply (*Ha! If only it were simple!*) notice that carrying a grudge is unskillful and unwise. To believe that getting mad somehow helps me is an error in thinking and is entirely human. People all around us—in movies and politics, for instance—normalize these unskillful mind-states, so naturally we think that it's okay to express our irritation-filled opinions. Our national political figures seem to revel in the contagious mind-states of fear and anger. We have to be very careful not to catch them ourselves. That's the reason I quarantine myself from the national news—news stations are often selling fear and even hatred. I don't need to buy into that.

When various friends begin their own political rants—of whatever stripe—I try not to reinforce their behavior by nodding my head or saying, "Unh-hunh." I may drift away to the bathroom or to washing the dishes. Leaving the conversation is easier if it's not a one-on-one monologue.

"Your worst enemy cannot harm you as much as your own unguarded thoughts," says the Buddha. Those unguarded thoughts are rat poison for me.

No Fear

I SAY I HAD no fear of cancer and no fear during diagnosis, surgery, and treatment. By this time, dear reader, you've read far enough to judge for yourself whether I am telling the truth . . . or whether fear was hiding from me.

I don't think I am afraid of death. During one month-long retreat, I went to bed and dreamed that Death was in bed with me. At first, I felt terrified, and then I felt compassionate toward Death. I even felt love toward Death.

Like all of us, I fear the death of the self, the death of ego, because then where will "I" be? To this end, I work to deconstruct the self every day, so that the self is undermined and turns out to be nothing more than a bubble. *Pop!*

I can tell you when fear did show up, unexpectedly. I received a phone call from my biggest stressor. We didn't talk long, and my body was overcome with what I thought was fury. I could taste adrenalin, feel my heart pounding as if all my blood was racing through my upper chest. And then I realized that this was not fury. My stressor had said nothing to make me angry. This full-on body response was fear. That's how afraid I am of my stressful person.

I have long known that, theoretically, underneath anger is fear or sadness. The moment after the phone call was the first time that I experienced how fear and anger feel the same in the body. I revisited that feeling of fear in the body several times that day, sinking into the uncomfortable sensations in the body, the feeling of tightness in the chest and the challenge of trying to keep the mind at bay while I soaked in the feeling of fear. I was hoping that a word or two might bubble to the surface of consciousness, so that the mind could understand this fear. *Bully* was the only word that occurred to me. Oh. This fear, this full-on body response is what being bullied feels like. Soon after, the feeling dissipated until I couldn't feel it or access it any longer.

The antidote to fear and the antidote to anger are the same: kindness. I consider this investigation of fear to be a kindness to myself. No need to resist this unpleasant feeling. No need to push it away. No need to project anger onto my stressful person. Let the fear live until it dies its natural death, and the bubble of fear pops. Notice that fear arises, and it passes away. It comes and goes. I don't need to hang onto fear and identify myself as a fearful person. I don't need to believe that the other person is a bully. There are moments when s/he acts like a bully, and other moments when s/he doesn't.

My challenge is to act in accordance with the loving-kindness sutta and be "straightforward and gentle in speech," instead of constantly trying to please the bully so s/he will be happy for a moment.

In fact, now that I've seen/felt this relationship as a bullying one, I can decide to step away from this dear person. I don't really need to keep "bullying" them (in my mind) to be a different person, a kinder person, or the person I want them to be.

I can simply step aside and let them go on about their life without me.

Don't Project a Self onto Others

ONE OF THE many intriguing things that Ayya Khema says is "Don't project a self onto others." What does that mean?

I think I understand it, intellectually. If I don't have a self, then no one else does either. Yet I go through my every day projecting a self onto others, assuming they have agency, as I think, *If only he wouldn't do that* or *If only she would realize such-and-such*. The self is an assumption we begin to make when we are about three years old. We never question that assumption.

What we call the self is just a collection of impersonal processes unrolling. But that's not how it feels. It feels to me as if I have free will, as if I'm the boss of my self, yet that's not what brain studies show. My decision to respond is made a tenth of a second before I become aware of it. It happens, then "I" become aware of it, and "I," the ego, claims responsibility for it, as if it were all "my" doing. But really, it's impersonal processes unrolling. As Andrew Olendzki quips, "We don't have free will. We have free won't."

I've puzzled over this piece of wisdom, about not projecting a self onto others, which remains elusive, but now I have the Cheryl Corollary: *Don't project* MY *self onto other people.* Of course, I do it all the time. Everything, and I mean everything, is projection. Although I have glimpsed this insight several times, I often forget it. Every feeling and every quality that I ascribe to another person is actually my own.

If people don't believe me when I say I had no fear, (a) they could be right, and (b) they might be projecting their own fear onto me.

Projection is a tricky little bugger. We usually project our worst qualities onto someone else, some handy person standing nearby—perhaps standing near our heart. You can often see this in the "problem child" of a family. Someone has to carry the shadow; someone has to balance the family's strong suit. That would be the problem child, the one who just doesn't measure up, because they're playing a discordant note in the symphony of the family.

We project our worst qualities or our negative qualities onto someone else, and then we get mad at them for having those qualities. Ingenious, isn't it? In lieu of being mad at ourselves, we get mad at another person. The ego protects itself at every turn. *Not me. Not me. Unh-uh. No, siree. It's her!* (The ego points the finger of projection.) *She's the problem! It's all her fault. Blame her.*

I would much rather blame someone else. When I feel that I've been blamed myself, I nearly suffocate under the wrongness of it.

Once in a while I try to silently reinterpret what someone says to me by substituting a different pronoun. When they say "you," in my mind, I try to hear it as "I."

Don't project a self onto others reminds me to pause when a friend doesn't believe I had no fear. "How could you not be afraid of cancer?"

"You could be right," I smile.

Where Is Bill?

SOMETHING SEEMS TO be missing in these pages, and that something is Bill. "Where is Bill?" you may ask.

Bill is there in the daily chitchat of life. Bill is there maintaining the house, making sure the woodshed is full of wood and that the snow is shoveled off the front step and the back walk. Bill is at the dinner table, waiting for me to cook something up, and then he's cleaning up the kitchen afterwards. I come down to a clean kitchen every morning. And because Bill is the last one out of bed, he makes the bed.

I straighten up the main floor—the kitchen, the dining room, and the living room. I corral his ADHD tendencies of far-flung papers—junk mail, bills, receipts, and three days' worth of newspapers—into his corner of the kitchen table. (Meanwhile, my office and sewing room upstairs are cluttered with dozens of my unfinished projects.) He retreats to his music studio downstairs for hours every day to practice piano, or to watch various serials of spies or cops and robbers on Roku at ten at night. We have an ordinary household relationship flavored by our own particularities. We cohabit comfortably.

I sometimes call Bill "Tigger" as he bounces into activity or into enthusiastically meeting the next new person. It turns out that Tiggers have two speeds: high and off. My Tigger needs quite a bit of down time in order to sproing into action. When he's on "high," he doesn't have time to sit with me and listen for an hour. He needs to go practice the piano for his concert. He needs to do his physical therapy exercises or take a hike or go biking. A vague discomfort in his body drives him to activity, while I stay comfortably at home, curled up on the sofa, writing. When he's "off," he is loafing downstairs in his man-cave music studio.

He probably has a hard time thinking of me as needy, since I'm the bossy big sister who does most of the organizing. He's the youngest brother, the one who is constantly relating to everyone around him as he tries to put people into a good mood.

Bill is my one-and-only, but he is not my one and only support person. I rely on Bill to keep the home fires burning (literally); I rely on other friends to go to the doctor with me (Barbara), to figure out treatment options (other survivors), and to talk through my feelings (my morning meditation group). I rely on Bill for hugs and for holding me in the middle of the night. I rely on him for companionship and some good laughs. I've written a hundred stories about Bill and his pratfalls—I am always the straight man to his funny man, Abbott to his Costello. Bill enjoys playing the role of the fool. "For I am a bear of very little brain," he says, quoting Winnie-the-Pooh.

While fools can be surprisingly wise, I find there are times when Bill does not give me the best advice. Our nearest and dearest sometimes unconsciously put their own needs and wishes ahead of our own. As any family therapist will tell you, a family system resists change.

For instance, several years ago, Bill and I had a trip to the Grand Canyon planned when my brother called to say that Dad's health was failing. I couldn't decide whether to cut out the trip to the Grand Canyon or delay going to see my dad. Bill said, "Let's go on to the Grand Canyon, as we had planned." My good friend said, "Go see your Dad." I went with Bill to the Grand Canyon for a week, then went to see my dad for the last six days of his life. It all worked out fine. But if I had it to do over again, I would skip the Grand Canyon.

For everyday decisions, I rely on Bill's advice, but when it comes to life-changing events, I rely on my women friends.

And so, in the telling of my story of cancer, Bill is there, taking out the compost and avidly recycling everything he can lay his hands on; he even goes dumpster-diving in our neighborhood trash receptacle in order to recycle what the neighbors have thrown away. Every evening he is busy telling me about his day. He tells me everything—his innermost secrets of whom he flirted with, his libido, his elimination system. Aries rising means he has no filters. I receive the raw, unedited version of his life and count myself lucky to have found such a faithful and candid companion.

Bill is the Sherpa on my journey through cancer. He takes care of base camp, but he is not planning the next step of my journey with me. I go to the doctor or to radiation with one or another of my friends. The cancer is no big deal to him; he's sure I can manage it, and that our life together will soon resume its natural course.

Bill does not make transitions easily, so it is taking time for him to shift his view of me. He wants the Cheryl I was four months ago, not this Cheryl who is putting his needs second or third or last.

He nags me to do this or that household chore. He's right, it should be done; meanwhile, I dilly-dally on making a phone call or sewing on a button for him or finishing one of my dozen projects. It, whatever *it* is, still doesn't get done. Since I appear to be as busy as usual, just when, exactly, am I going to stay home and take care of my share of the chores? "Not this month," I tell him, and he exhales a huffing breath. "When?" he demands. "I don't know," I say, trying to be honest.

My straightforwardness was one of the qualities that attracted him when we met. "You're not complicated," he said. He had just escaped a marriage to a complicated woman.

I am also low-maintenance. I spent twenty years as a single woman, so I can take care of myself. Bill and I each roll along in our own directions, held together by some marvelous universal joint that keeps us in tandem even though we travel at different speeds and in different gears. Bill and I do not share the same spiritual path. He is as interested in my meditation as I am in his music. It's beautiful, but my eyes glaze over when his conversation with his musical friends turns to dominant sevenths and major thirds. He, in turn, doesn't even ask me about my meditation. I know the Dharma has affected him, and that is enough. He is not a spiritual seeker, and I am.

Nevertheless, we often talk about what one of us will do when the other is gone. Bill, who is a church organist, calls God his Companion. In his solitary activities, Bill never walks alone. He often thanks his Companion for the blessings of his life.

I thank Bill for being my companion on my life's journey.

Wake Up to Dying

T HE WAKE UP to Dying project came to Brattleboro in the spring. The displays and art projects in a
downtown building were open every day for three days,
with panels of speakers featured every late afternoon and
evening.

The local hospice asked me to sit on the spiritual
panel along with a Congregationalist minister and a
Jewish storyteller. We each began by talking about our
own spiritual traditions around death. I wanted to go last,
since Buddhism has a different focus.

The Protestant minister talked about the richness of
Catholic rituals, such as last rites, final communion, and
wakes, while she felt her own tradition has not empha-
sized rituals as much.

We all agreed that the Jewish tradition has a host of
wonderful rituals. The body of the deceased is washed
by a committee of community members to purify it, and
then it is wrapped in a plain linen shroud. The casket,
a plain wooden coffin, remains closed after the body is
wrapped. As a sign of respect, the body is watched over
from the time of death till burial. The kaddish, a prayer in
honor of the dead, is said. The family sits shiva for a week

after the death of a loved one, and may tear their clothes or wear a black ribbon. Then, a year later, a Jahrzeit candle is lit to mark the anniversary of the death.

Buddhism, however, directs our meditation toward what are called the three characteristics of all experience: impermanence, unsatisfactoriness, and not-self. When we see that everything is constantly changing, we become aware of a niggling feeling of dissatisfaction. Wonderful things come to an end, but we want more; we want them to continue. Difficult things visit us, and we want them to go away.

When we see that everything is constantly changing, then we can begin to glimpse how nothing in the world exists permanently. Our language gives us categories, so we speak in categories and concepts as a way to deal with this constant flux. I call my garden "garden," even though it changes in so many ways throughout the day. The word *garden* makes me think of it as something solid, something unchanging, something that permanently "exists." The same ever-changing flux of the garden applies to the word *Cheryl*. I'm definitely not the same Cheryl I was a few months ago, or even yesterday. Slowly, we begin to see that our idea of our self as an unchanging, fixed self (or Self) is purely imaginary. Not even we, ourselves, exist for more than a moment before something changes—we breathe, we blink, our heart beats, we change our mind— and we have a new existence. Life is like frames in the film of a movie, changing many times a second—so fast that we have the illusion of continuity and solidity. We are being born and dying every minute, every second.

What, then, is "death" but one more of the millions of mini-deaths we have already experienced—if we were paying attention. The ego, of course, rebels against this idea, because what we are really saying here is "death to the ego," and the ego wants to *live*, at all costs.

Buddhism walks the Middle Way between eternalism (believing that we have undying souls) and annihilationism (the scientific materialism that says, "When you die, it's all over").

In meditation, we can sometimes see that "our" stream of consciousness is actually impersonal, simply flowing on, impelled by ignorance and craving and habit (also called karma). Though the process is impersonal, the illusion of personality continues to be quite strong as we claim our particular collection of habits and sensations (this moment's collection, anyway) as "me" and "mine."

Buddhist practice offers many contemplations aimed at deconstructing the self. The most accessible contemplation is one that the Buddha invited us to reflect on every day, the five daily reflections:

> *I am of the nature to grow old.*
> *I am of the nature to become ill.*
> *I am of the nature to die.*
> *Everything I cherish will change and vanish.*
> *Karma is the only thing I own.*

Needless to say, these reflections are not very popular, and they are real conversation-stoppers.

I could feel that the energy in the room had sagged during my five-minute talk, so I stopped expounding. As I said, the ego is quite disinclined to hear about such things as looking life—or death—straight in the eye.

Most of the questions from the audience were aimed at the Christian minister and the engaging Jewish storyteller. Then a blonde woman raised her hand and told her story. She was visiting from out of town. Thirty years earlier she had married a Mormon and converted. She totally bought into all the Mormon beliefs and was very happy with her faith. A year before this gathering, she had had outpatient surgery. Apparently, she was allergic to the anesthetic, because everything went black, and she felt she was going to die. By this point in telling the story she was in tears, and her friend sitting next to her put her hand on the woman's leg. "Everything I believed in," the blonde woman said, "wasn't there. I felt terrified."

The Christian and the Jew groped for their responses, so I said, "Terror is a step on the spiritual path." Since no one asked me to explain exactly what this means, I didn't.

Shortly afterward our discussion came to an end, and the blonde Mormon came over to hug me. As I drifted toward the door, a friend said to me, "I was surprised to hear that terror is a step on the spiritual path." I smiled and nodded my head.

If you're not expecting it, the first glimpse into the no-thing-ness of not-self, or no-ego, is indeed terrifying.

You might experience it the first time you hear the word *cancer* pointed straight at your body.

Suddenly it's time, whether you want to or not, to wake up to dying.

THE NEW ME:
Oncology

Nipple

WHEN I WAS twenty-five, in the summer of 1973, I stopped wearing a bra. To hide my nipples when I was in public, I covered each one with a band-aid so that the T-shirt clinging to my breasts wouldn't show my nipples.

That little bump was lost to view.

Ten years ago, my cousin Jeana sent an e-mail to all her women friends and relatives, warning them to beware of inverted nipples because they were a symptom of invasive breast cancer. My right nipple had begun to invert at times, then pop out again, but the doctor didn't seem concerned. This went on for about five years, until it finally went into hiding and wouldn't come out of seclusion. Not even hot nights with my lover could coax it out to play. Naked coldness could not force it out to shiver with its mate. No, it stayed inside, inverted, introverted—nice and warm and cozy.

I rather liked its smooth appearance pressing firmly against my form-fitting Smartwool sweaters. One smooth breast, one nippled breast. Occasionally I felt self-conscious about being naked and getting into the hot tub at night with a friend, but, hey, it was dark.

She couldn't really see me that well without her glasses anyway.

Since my doctor wasn't concerned, I thought nothing about it. Then in 2014, I asked the mammogram technician to show me what was pulling the nipple inward. Something sticky perhaps? But eight years of x-rated rays revealed no culprit, despite my breasts being scrunched between those cold metal plates on the big pink machine that I hugged to my chest once a year.

My body functioned perfectly well with this imperfection.

Toward the end of seven weeks of radiation, the inverted nipple oozed a few drops of a clear plasma, which produced a small, bloodless scab. It itched. Radiation can itch. Occasionally, I felt tiny pings and imagined that adhesions were letting go. And then, one month after radiation ended, my right nipple popped out of its hiding place. At first, it didn't look like a twin to the other one, but gradually, over the course of a few weeks, my right nipple was back in play. The areola was ever so slightly bluish from the blue dye injection on the day of surgery.

None of the doctors ventures an opinion about why this happened. The radiologist, the surgeon, my primary care physician—they all shrug. But the surgeon tells me my now-extroverted radiated breast will look younger and more sprightly than its twin. He's right.

Canceling the Scheduled Vacations

BILL AND I had planned to go hiking in the Lake District in England around the summer solstice. That vacation had to be canceled because I wasn't done with radiation. Then we were going to go to a lake resort in northern Vermont to float in the water and read books after my radiation, but that had to be canceled, too. And thereby hangs a tale.

While I was on my four-day retreat in Virginia, three days after radiation ended, Bill slipped while hiking with a friend and ruptured the quadriceps tendon on his right knee. He was carried off the mountain in a toboggan by ten EMTs; he had emergency knee surgery the next day. Since I was in cyber-silence, I knew nothing about his adventure until thirty hours after a neighbor had brought him home from the hospital in a locked knee brace with plenty of pain medication.

Bill is a somatic guy; his emotions are acted out in his body. Fourteen years earlier, Bill had had a trip to the hospital while I was on retreat—he broke four ribs while cross-country skiing. His body was saying what he could not bring himself to say out loud. *Don't abandon me. I'm afraid my rib-woman will break our relationship, leave me, and go meditate for the rest of her life.* Consciously, he was trying to be a big boy and act like it was okay for me to leave him at home for a week. However, his unconscious was acting like a little boy, the baby boy who came home from the hospital six months before his depressed mother did. His father hired a nurse to be with infant Billy 24/7, and the nurse loved him completely. When his mother came home six months later, the nurse left. No wonder this man has abandonment issues! Had Bill fallen on one knee, begging me not to abandon him? *"Don't go! Don't go!"*

For the next five weeks after Bill ruptured his quadriceps tendon, I chauffeured him everywhere he needed to go. I'd never been to his doctor's appointments with him before. I had never waited an hour while he had his physical therapy appointments. I had never before run all his errands for him. As any caregiver can tell you, each trip to town took twice as much time as I expected it to. I was surprised by how much patience I had.

I was at Bill's beck and call. And I am *not* by nature Nurse Jane Fuzzy-Wuzzy. Every morning and every night, I put ice packs on his knee and calf and then cinched up his leg brace to keep the packs in place. Every evening, I washed his right leg after he had given himself a sponge bath. Every night he peed into quart jars while lying in bed with his leg brace on; every morning I watered my flowerpots with his urine. The flowers by my front door had never looked so fantastic.

I drove him to our neighbors' pool-in-a-pasture every afternoon so he could swish his leg in water and then, eventually, swim.

Bill cursed himself for ruining his summer with a moment of mindlessness. One misstep off the mountain trail meant no hiking and practically no walking. No biking except for the exercise bicycle at the physical therapist's office. For five weeks, he could not play the organ, which has a foot-pedal keyboard, nor could he use the pedal on his piano. But he did gain one thing: my complete attention and companionship for five weeks.

Somatic Me

So if Bill is a somatic guy, how am I a somatic gal? How is my body saying something that my mind doesn't particularly want to hear? What is cancer waking me up to in my life? What have I been asleep to?

My friend Nancy calls breast cancer a cosmic sledgehammer. She knew there were changes she needed and wanted to make in her life. Breast cancer was her wake-up call to follow her bliss. It took her six years to change tracks. Six years to extract herself from her struggling law practice and find the international career she had been yearning for. Her first step was to volunteer for a year with the American Bar Association in the Republic of Georgia. With that experience on her resume, she was on her way to working around the globe.

Now it's time to pause and assess *my* life. I wouldn't call cancer a sledgehammer, but it certainly is a wake-up call.

If cancer is doubling in size every year and eating up everything in sight, then I want to explore the question "What's eating me?"

What's eating me? I know the answer to that question in a heartbeat. It's my most difficult relationship. It's time to stop placating the bully in my life and start practicing tough love. I need to stop my enabling behavior, stop my bend-over-backwards behavior, stop my trying-to-be-helpful behavior. The most helpful thing for me would be for this difficult person to stop browbeating me. Therefore, I need to stop walking on eggshells and speak straightforwardly *and* gently to this person.

Making this change is not easy, and it goes against my nice-girl tendencies to keep the peace. But keeping the outer peace riles up my mind so much that my inner peace is deeply disturbed. I've had to set bottom lines with an addict in my life before, and this feels very similar.

How can I say "No" with an open heart? I don't have to fight. I don't have to get mad. I don't have to carry a grudge. I don't have to be hardhearted. I don't have to put on my armor to ward off this person's thoughtless zingers. All I have to do is step aside.

It turns out that we humans have two immune systems—one fights off viruses, bacteria, and unfamiliar cancer cells when we feel we are in a safe environment. This is where the body "rests and digests," or repairs itself. On the other hand, if we are threatened, the inflammatory response of the immune system is activated. But if we are in fight-or-flight mode due to chronic stress, despite there being no actual threat of physical injury, too many inflammatory-response cells go on the warpath; and they can begin to cause internal damage to the body and potentially even feed cancerous metastases.

If there's too much inflammation in my body, I might ask myself, in relationship to cancer: "What's my burning issue?" *What burns me?* has pretty much the same answer as *What's eating me?*

If I look closely, I can also see a very low-grade fever, a dull and distant twinge that's easy to ignore in my dear and loving relationship. Everyone makes some sort of sacrifice when they pair up with someone else. First of all, they take on the other person's karma. You'd think that your own karma would be sufficient for this one lifetime, but no. Blinded by love, we think it's going to be just him and me or her and me. As the years go on, the holidays and perhaps our various in-laws' idiosyncrasies begin to get on our nerves. Still, the benefits of our relationship outweigh those irritating in-laws or our partner's annoying habits. So we stick with this person. We've made our bed—maybe it's a fairly comfortable bed, most of the time—and we'll lie in it. The ongoing annoyance submerges itself in our subconscious, where we might see it if we cared to look, or maybe we're so unconscious of our discontent that our conscious mind denies its existence at all. Perhaps we forget what being true to our self means. We're being true-blue to this other person, but that little grain of sand of not being true to our self rubs us unconsciously. We carry a tension we don't even know we're carrying, and after a few decades, it might show up in the body.

Lydia, an evangelical, truly believes in submitting to her husband's rule of home and family. She developed a digestive problem. I wonder what she can't swallow or what she can't stomach in her relationship. A modern woman just cannot hand herself and all her decisions over to her husband, even though her mind totally believes in doing so. The body tells true.

I read a book by an American woman who converted to Islam and married an Egyptian. She loved her new religion and truly believed in it. Then, while living in Cairo, she developed such severe allergies that she had to move back to the United States. What else besides something in Cairo was she allergic to?

What, in my own relationship, have I submerged in order to smooth the coupled path?

For the first four years of my relationship with my sweetie, I stopped going to my weekly meditation group. "Oh, just stay home this evening with me," he would say. After a few months, I completely forgot about the weekly sitting group. Then I wanted to go on a weeklong retreat. "Oh, that's not a good time," he would say. "Maybe later." It took a few years for "later" to arrive, a few years before I stopped putting off my heart's desire. A few years before I valued that little voice in the background more than the pleasure of staying home and snuggling with my sweetie. The Buddha calls this reordering of priorities forgoing a lesser, temporary pleasure for the greater mind-changing pleasure that meditation can bring.

So let me return to the question of what I have sacrificed in order to maintain the status quo of my own relationship. If I were single, I'd go on a three-month retreat this year. Most of the people who have been on these long retreats call them transformative. I feel very fortunate that my sweetie has agreed to and expects me to go on a one-month retreat every winter. Do I have the nerve to up the ante and take the fallout, whatever that might be? Do I have the courage to be true to myself?

If I'm not true to myself, no one else is going to do it for me, not even my true love. In fact, our loved ones are rather comfortable with the status quo; change is uncomfortable. When it comes right down to it, our dearly beloved are more interested in their own comfort than in ours. It's up to me to initiate the change to be true to myself.

My body has given me the message of cancer. I don't expect to be able to fully decode this message for another ten years or so. In the meantime, I try to decipher the clues that cancer offers: What's eating me? What inflames me? What little bit of hidden irritation (in my closest relationships) might have calcified, and how can I turn that rough grain of sand into a luminescent pearl of wisdom?

After all, life is short. I'm keenly aware of that, now that cancer has woken me up to my beautiful life, no matter how long it is—or isn't.

What's Important

A MEDITATION STUDENT (it could be me) complains to her meditation teacher that her meditation practice has slipped. There are so many other things to do. The meditation master takes a jar and fills it up with rocks.

"Can I add more?" he asks.

"Well, no-o-o," says the student doubtfully.

He picks up a handful of gravel and shakes it down into the jar among the rocks. "Can I add some more?" he asks again.

"Hmmm," she responds.

He takes some smaller pebbles and adds those to the jar, shaking them down between the gravel. "Can I add more?" he asks.

The student is silent.

He takes a handful of sand and shakes that down between the pebbles, the gravel, and the rocks.

"So what's the lesson here?" he asks the student.

She sighs. "That I can always add one more thing."

"No," says the meditation teacher. "Put the big rocks in first."

So what are my big rocks?—and especially now that I've caught a glimpse of illness from cancer, and the fast track of aging via the anti-cancer drug I take. Maybe I have even glanced at death in the rear-view mirror. So what's most important? What's really, really important?

My spiritual development is number one for me. Nowadays, most activities have to pass through the screen of *Does this augur well for my long-term well-being?*

Gail, who recently turned seventy after a rocky ride through her sixties that included cancer, says she sometimes picks up a magazine and then thinks, *I've only got ten more years. I don't have time to read this magazine*, and she puts it down again. Gail joined the Catholic Church as part of her spiritual development. She's a people person and enjoys the community that a church provides.

To begin with, my ego fills my weekly calendar with plays, lectures, concerts, and volunteer activities. In actuality, these scheduled activities are plans for the person I want to be, the person I want to become—more knowledgeable, more cultural, more sociable. My ego is my social planner. On the day of the event, I look at my calendar again, through the screen of my spiritual welfare. No, I'm not going to that movie. No, I'm not going to that play. No, I'm not going to that very interesting wildlife lecture. Having a quiet life turns out to be more important than having a busy life.

As you might expect, one of my big rocks is daily meditation and going on retreat—a one-month retreat every year, plus four or six week-long retreats, plus half a dozen day-long retreats. My reading is almost limited to Dharma books; I read very few works of fiction. Occasionally I have an all-Dharma day—three or four activities that all include some aspect of the Dharma. These are really good days.

I enjoy teaching the Dharma, because teaching deepens my own understanding of the Buddha's teachings. Sometimes I find myself saying things in class or in a Dharma talk that I didn't know I knew. Teaching the Dharma gives me joy. *Dharma* is sometimes translated as "the nature of things." Living the Dharma every day feels like being in accord with nature.

Another of my big rocks is Bill. Companionship with Bill is one of the great gifts of my midlife. Now that we are walking, or, in his case, hobbling toward the next stage of life, our relationship is changing ever so slightly, as aging creeps in on little cat feet. Our traveling days are not exactly over, but maybe it's time to go to one place and stay there for a week or two instead of touring around.

Bill and I have long been accustomed to our own independence and our mutual interdependence, but soon, perhaps too soon, we will be depending on each other for our physical well-being. The time may be coming when I no longer meditate/read/teach the Dharma, but instead simply live the Dharma through my relationship to Bill.

Another big rock is service to my community. Being of service is in my bones. I began my adult life by being a Volunteer In Service To America—a VISTA volunteer—when I was twenty-two. I remain a volunteer in service to the dying and the bereaved through hospice, to the homeless at the Overflow Shelter, to my neighborhood by being a helpful neighbor, to the town I live in through the Dummerston Community Chest and Prospect Hill park, to local gardeners as a Master Gardener and Master Composter. In fact, I'm also in service to the whole world through my philanthropy. This year, I have, unexpectedly, been of service to the New England Center for Circus Arts by performing my trapeze routine at two of their fund-raisers as they work toward raising $2 million for the first purpose-built trapezium in this country.

I'd like to focus on offering daily service to anyone who crosses my path. I'm particularly inspired by a Dharma friend, Lynn, who lives in Australia and writes a blog on the five ethical precepts of doing no harm. When I see her once a year, she is remarkably thoughtful and caring—a learned behavior, I'm sure, since she's a strong personality, a leader in any situation. Can I practice being warm, gentle, and thoughtful?

Writing is still one of my big rocks, though my annual reflection books may be winding down. I made a commitment to writing after my dad died, after I stopped working full-time. First of all, I think of writing as a form of teaching the Dharma. Secondly, I think of writing as reinforcing my ego, as trying desperately to shore up my self by working on this immortality project of writing out my life. Thirdly, I think of writing as my talent. (Mercury, the planet of communication, conjunct with Jupiter, the really big planet of luck and good fortune, which is also conjunct with my Sun—that would be me at the center of my universe—in my third house of communication.) At any rate, I'm not ready to place writing on a lower shelf just yet.

Dharma, Bill, service, and writing. These are the big rocks of my daily life. Putting these big rocks of my daily life first keeps me attuned to the mission of my life— waking up and living generously and compassionately. These are the qualities that give meaning to my life. I could call it living consciously.

Gardening, which used to be a big rock, has moved down a notch. I still enjoy my gardens tremendously, of course. I love talking about flowers and vegetables and landscaping. As a Master Gardener and Master Composter, I give talks in the community every two or three months about various aspects of gardening. And, for heaven's sake, I write a gardening blog!* During the time of my diagnosis, I was just finishing writing a book, *The Real Dirt on Composting*. But if the truth be told, as much fun as that book was to write, I'm not really interested in writing non-Dharma material.

I no longer garden psychically—I don't carry my garden in my psyche as parents do their children or as some people do their dogs or cats. I no longer buy rare plants or mail-order specialty plants. I used to desire to have one of everything in my garden. Now I see that

---

* www.themeditativegardener.blogspot.com.

certain plants love to grow in my garden—often they are plants I would not have chosen, like mullein. So I collect varieties of what wants to grow in my backyard, and have stopped fighting for the lives of all the plants that limp along. I finally understood this after collecting hundreds of white plastic markers of plants that had died.

Seeing the impermanent nature of the garden and everything in it (e.g., another garden bench broke), I feel more dispassionate about the springing up and falling apart of the garden. Gardening gladdens my heart, and I am surrendering my garden to Life.

When I was a young adult, my dad told me I had sand in my shoes. He was right: I wanted to travel the world, and many friends think that this is exactly what I've done. Still, I've "only" been to about fifty countries and all fifty states. Although I do enjoy traveling, I've become less excited about it, partly because I see the impermanent nature of the sights I see. I visit a marvelous World Heritage site one day, probably for a few hours. I buy a postcard. I take photos. And then it all drops into my memory bank. Money spent, time spent, and then it's gone, and I am face to face with my daily life again. The memory of those glorious weeks is now reduced to sound bites with friends whose attention is distracted by incoming texts and e-mails, or who detour the conversation onto what they were just reminded of. No one really has time to truly listen to me relate the joys of my journey—and why should they? The past, even the recent past, is as dry as dust. Only this very moment is alive. In this respect, travel has turned into sand running between my fingers.

I now have a mortal view of travel: I want to travel to see or spend time with loved ones. Our time together is precious. I no longer need to collect new places for my travel résumé. I post my photos on Facebook, and people comment. Otherwise, my travel photos are of interest to no one else in the world but me.

I no longer take many photos at all because, really, who has time to look at them? I can post them to Facebook for one second of my friends' attention. Or, if I wanted to spend, say, five minutes per photo—naming, filing, uploading, printing—I could organize them into an album. Photos have turned into sand for me.

Our community, the Brattleboro area, has a rich arts life. For Bill, this continues to be one of the centerpieces of his life as he attends perhaps four musical events every weekend. I am very happy to have a date with him on Friday and Saturday nights and happy to see friends at plays or concerts or lectures, but if Bill really wants to go to one event that I do not, I am perfectly content to stay home or go to another event by myself.

Do I really want to spend my precious time on house maintenance? At age thirty-one, when I built my house, I looked forward to designing my very own environment. Mission accomplished. Now the house always needs maintaining. I don't resent maintenance, or the money spent on maintenance—the price I pay to live where I want to live.

Which brings me to the topic of my neighborhood. When I was thirty-one, I bought eighty acres of land cooperatively with six couples. We each built our own houses. All these years later, there have been two deaths and three divorces. Mostly it is the women who have remained in our little community on a dead-end dirt road in the woods. So when I refer to "my morning meditation group," I am talking about people I have known for more than forty years. My little community of neighbors is the bedrock of my daily life.

Being embedded in a community contributes to longevity. We are now talking about "aging in place"—staying in our homes for as long as possible, with the support of each other as well as various community services.

What's most important to me is love, compassion, gratitude, generosity, being of service, fulfilling my talent, my relationships, and spending time outdoors.

Bill's purpose in life is to bring joy to people in the moment and make them smile. By looking people in the eye and smiling, even at store clerks whom he will never see again in his life, he receives a dose of oxytocin, the bonding chemical. He tries to crack their exterior presentation of business-as-usual to leave a wake of warm feelings behind so that people feel good about themselves. This intention liberates shy people (e.g., *moi*) and allows them to do what needs to be done. As Maya Angelou said, "People will forget what you said. People will forget what you did. But people will not forget how you made them feel."

When I am on my deathbed, I don't want to regret my unlived life. I want to have taken this once-in-a-lifetime opportunity to hear, see, feel, taste, and smell the life that surrounds me. So it's important *now* for me to spend more time in solitude, more time in service to people, more time outdoors in nature, more time in Dharma practice, more time loving life and loving the people I see every day. These are the rocks upon which I build my life.

Not-Important

OUR LOCAL HOSPICE has a choir called Hallowell, which sings at the bedsides of dying people. When the director, Kathy Leo, was teaching a hospice choir workshop in Providence, Rhode Island, one of the participants told her that, although she never remembers her dreams, her recently deceased sister came to her in a dream and said, "You'd be surprised by the number of things that don't matter."

Even before my cancer diagnosis, I'd been contemplating "important" and "not important," but this heavenly messenger of disease renews my attention to the subject.

You may be familiar with the time-management matrix offered by Stephen Covey in his book *Seven Habits of Highly Effective People.*

	URGENT	NOT URGENT
IMPORTANT		• Exercise • Planning for...
NOT IMPORTANT	• Interruptions such as... • Distractions such as...	• Time wasters such as...

Take a moment now to jot down a few things that are important and not important for you.

On my laundry list of what's not-important is shopping for more clothes. Really, I can only wear one pair of pants at a time, one pair of shoes at a time. I truly, truly already have enough clothes. Too many clothes, in fact.

Author Anne Lamott tells of going shopping with a friend who had just weeks to live. Anne tried on this little black dress and that one, asking her friend's opinion. Finally, her friend said, "Anne. You don't have that kind of time." None of us has that kind of time.

Not only do I want to stop collecting clothes, I am really trying to put the brakes on collecting any more stuff at all, unless it's biodegradable. I have reviewed my various collections. All my garden paraphernalia could go to the Swap Program at the landfill tomorrow—except that I'm still using the flowerpots, the six-packs, the trays, the vases, the forcing vases. I distribute my small collection of heirlooms to my nieces and nephews as it occurs to me, though I do still have a dozen of my mother's paintings. Bill and I have agreed—our walls are full. I also have a closet that's half full of wall art. I believe that's called "too much." A ninety-two-year-old hospice client recently said to me, "Why did I waste my time collecting all this stuff?" She had a cabinet full of porcelain angels. "I don't care about this stuff. And my kids can have my money. I just don't care."

My collection of Christmas decorations has bitten the dust. I used to spend two days decorating and two days after Christmas undecorating. That's a lot of time spent on a holiday I don't really celebrate. I am now content with a small tree and a string of lights. The winter solstice festival, by whatever name, is really about light and dark anyway.

My cousin Nancy, who died twenty years ago, collected windmills—a collection now scattered to the winds. My mother collected angels. Also, gold slippers (fourteen pairs), batteries in case of a tornado (two shoeboxes full), and many other things in case the Great Depression returned tomorrow. Collections—of anything—come and go.

I recently saw a cartoon in which one character says to the other, "My desire to be well-informed is at odds with my desire to remain sane." Actually, my desire for sanity has trumped being well-informed. Since I neither listen to the news, watch the news, nor read the news, it is truly amazing how much news I pick up by osmosis. Really, what's the assumption behind being a newshound? That we are the watchdogs of democracy? That if we are well-informed, our personal opinions can change the course of world events?

Many of the news channels seem to be selling fear. Since I want to be careful about whom (and what) I spend my time with, I take my news in teaspoonfuls—one or two minutes at a time.

I stopped watching TV when I was nineteen. That's almost half a century ago. In her book *Animal, Vegetable, Miracle*, the story of her year as a locavore, Barbara King-solver writes about her teenage daughter begging her for a television. The mother tells her daughter to write down the list of what she's going to give up every day in order to watch TV: homework, chores, friends, exercise, creative projects, reading. Of course, her daughter cannot make a convincing case. I, too, cannot figure out what I would give up to have time to watch television, videos, or any other media.

Not-important includes Facebook and all the other social media that I can waste hours on. Facebook (Pinterest, Instagram, etc.) makes me feel related to people I love and people I know and acquaintances I just barely remember. I click the Like button to say, "Yoo-hoo. I'm here. I received your message. I care."

According to evolutionary psychologist Robin

Dunbar, we, as humans, are capable of maintaining five intimate relationships (our close support group, perhaps including family) plus about ten more good friends. Add another thirty-five people you'd invite over for dinner, and then another hundred, for a total of 150, that you'd invite to a party. That's it. That's the number of people we can really care about. Even with social-media connections to, perhaps, thousands of "friends," people actually feel lonelier and less connected than ever before. What really connects us is meaningful conversations and giving the gift of our presence.

While many people think of reading, puzzles, and games as relaxing, I think of these pastimes as escapes—diversions to make time pass pleasantly. I'm trying to escape a vague sense of emptiness in my life, and so I fill it up with these various momentary pleasant distractions.

I try not to let Sudoku or crossword puzzles cross my threshold. As one friend said, "Sudoku is like heroin to the vein." I'm addicted, so I try to stay Sudoku-sober at home. Sudoku or other puzzles can turn into time-wasters because the thrill of solving problems outweighs the mundane tasks I need to do or the twenty-minute meditation I have vowed to sit. *Oh, later*, I think. As you know, "later" never comes. However, just in case Sudoku is good for the brain, I do allow myself to do Sudoku on airplanes or while traveling—vacation times when I am definitely looking for escapes from the present moment. Puzzles may improve my memory—or not. More than exercising brain power, I want to practice using the power of the mind to reshape itself with admirable qualities such as patience and kindness. I want to rewire my brain and replace my irritable tendencies with openheartedness. That's the kind of brain exercise I want.

Reading can certainly expand my view of the world. Since I'm a lifelong learner, reading has been crucial to developing my nuanced views of the world. In high school, I read hundreds of the classics. In my twenties, I read fiction and all of Alice Bailey, a theosophist. In my thirties, I read history, Jungian psychology, and Native American literature. In my forties, I read psychology and nonfiction. Since age fifty, I've focused on the Dharma, with brief forays into any of the other subjects above. Yet, as a deaf friend said, "In one eye and out the other." It comes. It goes. I can't hang on to any of it—not the brain power nor the facts nor the thrill of solving a puzzle nor the memory of having read a book, let alone recalling what the plot was. I aim to avoid using reading as an escape; I just don't have that kind of time. Instead, I use reading for inspiration, information-gathering, or enlarging my world view.

What else is not-important? All the ego-maintenance projects that plump up our self-importance—more money, more status, a more prestigious job, an expensive car. The ego is a vast hole that can never be filled. No matter how much we have, we still feel a certain lack. When someone asked John D. Rockefeller how much money was enough, he said, "Just a little more than I have." We keep trying to fill this vague emptiness with more and more stuff, but that strategy has never been effective. We are going to lose it all in the end, no matter what.

Worrying. Now *there's* a time-consuming project that is not only not-important, it's also useless and even harmful. Worry represents a huge amount of wasted time and energy. We can sleepwalk through our lives as the mind jumps forward into "and next," "and then," "what if" . . . or we can actually live in the present moment. The choice is yours. As Mark Twain said, "Some of the worst things in my life never happened."

All the self-hatred, lack of self-confidence, believing we are not good enough, feelings of unworthiness—these judgments, feelings, and put-downs of the self are useless and even harmful to our mental welfare. What's important is to practice self-compassion as the antidote to guilt, self-blame, self-judgments, and feelings of unworthiness.

In fact, any form of resentment, dislike, or grudge is fairly unimportant. While visiting friends and family in Indiana (the most northern Southern state), I heard several people say, "I *hate* Obama" or "I *hate* Hillary—I can't stand her." We can't simply hate and get away with it; we can't hate and expect to just waltz right through those pearly gates. Hating is not a free-of-charge emotion. Hatred begets hatred. Hatred pollutes our soul and stains our very being. Hatred is really not-important and is a true waste of our human potential

We—our egos—so much want to be right (and therefore, "they"—the other person—*must* be wrong!), we so much want to be recognized as the good guy, that we project all our own unskillful qualities onto another person. I suppose this is the only way we can have an argument with ourselves, but the problem is that we believe the projection. We believe that the other person is actually bad or stupid or hateable. By withdrawing our hatred of others, we come to love our very own selves. Hatred never ceases by hating someone; hatred only ceases by love.*

Looking back at my short list of the unimportant clutter in my life, I find I've listed the same five distractions that hinder progress in meditation, the same five blockages that obstruct my spiritual life. As listed by the Buddha, these are sense desire (clothes shopping, for instance), ill-will (hatred and judgmentalness), laziness (for example, paying more attention to the unimportant, nonurgent things that suck up my time and attention), worry and anxiety, and skeptical doubt ("Just this one little distraction, this one little escape or game, won't matter").

What "don't matter" in the long run of our precious life are the distractions, escapes, and busy clutter that seem so enticing, important, and pressing in the moment. I'm sure I'd still be surprised at how many things in my daily life aren't really that important and "don't matter" in the long view. I have to keep reminding myself of the distractions I am aware of, and I pause, sometimes in the middle of opening junk mail or trying to clean up my

---

* Hatreds never cease by hatred; they cease by non-hatred; this is the primeval law (*Dhammapada* 5).

(virtual) e-mail in-box. Pause and breathe and remember that my life is slip-sliding away.

E. B. White said: "Omit unnecessary words." We could say *Omit unnecessary importance.*

Next-of-Kin Committee

ANNE, AN EIGHTY-TWO-YEAR-OLD Quaker who lives alone, told me about a clearness committee of her friends that she has met with twice a year for the past fourteen years. These are the women she wants to have around her as she enters late old age and, eventually, dying. These are the friends who will help her make decisions or carry out her decisions for her.

A week later, Doreen, a meditation teacher, aged seventy, told me about her next-of-kin committee—a committee of her friends, whom she gets together with once a year, to talk about her wishes for her old, old age and dying. Having taken her mother into her home for the last five years of her mother's life, Doreen is keenly aware of the possibilities.

My actual next-of-kin live far away from me. My brother Beau is 900 miles away, in Indiana, and he's quite busy with the lives of his four adult children and his two granddaughters, who live nearby. My sister Dona lives 2,700 miles away in the Idaho panhandle, near her younger son. She babysits for her two grandsons a couple of times a week. In other words, my next-of-kin are far away and intently focused on their own next-of-kin.

I like the idea of this next-of-kin committee, and want to call a meeting of my own. My next-of-kin committee includes Connie, who holds my durable power of attorney for health care; Barbara, RN (retired nurse), who holds my power of attorney in legal matters; Claire, my local meditation teacher; and, of course, Bill. Maybe my sister could Skype in to the conversation, since she is the trustee of my living trust.

Over time, we can talk about best- and worst-case scenarios. What to do in the best case? And what to do in a worst-case scenario that might go on for years? I could talk about what makes my life worth living and how they will know when to pull the plug.

Maybe they can catalyze me to write some letters of instruction. I've written one to the trustee who holds my power of attorney, but there are a few others I have yet to pen. I also need to rewrite my obituary, which has been on file at the funeral home for twenty years.

When the time comes, I will depend on my next-of-kin committee to offer me the kindness of death.

Anastrozole

A<small>S OF EARLY</small> August, anastrozole is my new best friend. Five months after my surgery, I finally got to meet her. I had to jump through a few hoops, though. For one thing, I needed to get a new bone density scan, which took three weeks to schedule. The good news is that I haven't lost any height in the past four years. I chalk this up to doing trapeze and aerial yoga and spending some time each week hanging upside down and thereby stretching out my spine.

The disappointing news is that my bones have lost density and become a bit more porous. Although I am still well within the range of osteopenia, my score is now –1.5 instead of –1.4. The score of minus one is the cutoff for osteopenia; –2.5 is the borderline for osteoporosis.

Anastrozole (shall I call her Anastasia?) is surprisingly petite. A tiny white tablet, easy to swallow without water. Our date is bedtime. She sleeps beside me on my nightstand.

There are a hundred different kinds of breast cancer. I have a variety that is estrogen-positive. Estrogen makes my type of cancer grow. Anastrozole inhibits the estrogen receptors. Anastasia is taking me into super-menopause.

You'd think that a sixty-seven-year-old woman would already *be* in super-menopause. Hot flashes receded into occasional warm-ups several years ago. My hair is thinning, so I have bangs again, like I did as a young woman—not to hide my high forehead, but to cope with the thin wispy hair at the edges of my scalp. Last year I complained of my thinning hair, and now it's going to become even thinner. Oh, great. In fact, Anastasia talked me into a haircut. I finally lopped off my scraggly ponytail and sent it to Locks of Love. The halo of white hair on the crown of my head now shines down over the brown hair all around the edges.

From now on, Anastasia is going to press the gas pedal and accelerate menopause. Let's just say, accelerate aging. The side effects of anastrozole include hot flashes. Fifteen years ago, I found that the benefit of hot flashes was that they attuned my mind perfectly to the wavelength for meditation. Yes, there was that tropical heat wave happening in my body, but I now know that the side effect of joy is that it heats up my body. Even when I don't recognize the presence of joy *per se*, I can feel the penetration of heat and recognize that the static of the ordinary mind is about to give way to nowness.

Other side effects of anastrozole include joint pain. Since having frozen shoulders at age fifty-five, I've taken glucosamine-chondroitin daily for all my joints. My juices and lubricating oils have dried up. No amount of silicone lubrication can disguise the sandpaper of what used to be so smooth and gliding.

Weight gain. Thanks to regular exercise, I've finally dropped five pounds, and now the prediction is that I'll gain it back plus some more.

The most worrisome of the side effects of no estrogen is bone loss. If I'm going to prevent that, I have to focus on bone maintenance every day. I need to get serious about weight-bearing exercises. I'm on the waiting list for Building Strong Bones, the Tufts University exercise regimen for old ladies. The routine is boring, but the social networking in a small town is a lot of fun; you're in on the latest-breaking news about everyone's health, travels, and family.

Of course, walking is the easiest weight-bearing exercise. Although I'm a loner, I now have to break out of my shell and make walking dates with others to get myself out of the house. Bill is a good exerciser. You'd think I would have a ready-made walking date there, but we live in different time zones. He likes to walk in the morning; I like to walk in the afternoon.

The time of day is the real rub here. I like to have my mornings to myself. My biorhythm sinks in mid- to late afternoon, and that's the time for me to exercise. But so many women like to exercise early, and that's when many exercise classes are offered.

Oh, Anastasia, you whose name means resurrection, keep me on the beam of my intention. Your gift of small poison offers the healing remedy I seek.

I've heard a lot of bad things about anastrozole. Some friends say, "I'm surprised at you, Cheryl. Taking a drug like that. It's so bad for you." Many friends report that they could only bear the side effects for a few months or maybe a year, then their oncologist switched them to a different drug, and maybe a few months later to yet a different one. Backpacker Liz, in her mid-fifties, bailed out of her daily medication after three years; she couldn't take the body aches anymore. Her Oncotype DX score was lower than mine.

So far, so good. It's only been a few weeks, and I have almost five more years to go. By the time I'm seventy-two, I can stop my daily date with Anastasia. But in five years, I may be ten years older than I am now.

No matter. I am seeking the resurrection that so many other women have talked about. "I had breast cancer seventeen years ago" . . . "twenty years ago" . . . "twenty-seven years ago."

No matter how long our resurrection, it doesn't last forever. The body still grows old, develops its own ailments. The body is mortal. The body eventually dies. And then it decays, giving rise to a new resurrection of grass, sky, and lake. The me in me never really was here anyway. The me always is in the daily resurrection of new day and new sun. New now.

Oh, Anastasia, thank you.

Exercising

I HATE EXERCISING. Oh, I've got my reasons. As a child, I had severe asthma, including athletics-induced asthma. While other kids were running around, I was reading a book. While other kids were in the band or playing team sports, I was sick in bed. Exercising means breathing hard, and breathing hard feels like wheezing, and wheezing makes me feel that I am suffocating.

At age thirty-five, I took up jogging. I lived in Portland, Oregon, where everyone was jogging or running outdoors, no matter the rain, the damp, the occasional sun. It took me two months to work up to a mile. I'd stop running and walk the rest of the way home, panting. It took another three months to work up to two miles. In the course of a year, I experienced runners' high twice, but I just didn't feel how great running was, the way my friend Mary Beth did. She loved running, as she did playing tennis, squash, and all the racquet sports. In fact, she didn't feel at home in her own body till she had run it a couple of miles. I don't get antsy like that. I don't feel the need to move.

Eventually I joined Mary Beth in a 5K race across the brand-new I-205 bridge over the Columbia River.

My top speed was ten minutes per mile; she was a seven-minute-mile gal.

When I reported on this race in a phone call to my grandmother, she was overcome. "Oh, heavenly days, Cherdy K. I never thought I'd see the day when you would be running. Lordy. Lordy."

I gave up running soon after that, and took up crew. My friend Nancy, a student at the Lewis & Clark Law School, was on the 6:00 A.M. crew on the Willamette River, and they needed another person for the eight-oar boat. That fitted perfectly with my schedule of going to work at 7:00 A.M. at the J. A. Wiley flooring company, just a few blocks away. After only three months, I could do chin-ups, which I'd never been able to do before in my life.

Then I left Portland with its outdoorsy culture and returned to my sedentary ways at the end of a dirt road in Vermont. Three years later, I met Bill, a hiker and a bicycler. He soon had me huffing and puffing up hills and mountains. When we tested our air outflow on a spirometer, he could puff out twice as much as I could. At age forty-five, I had the lung power of an eighty-year-old woman. Still I persevered, doing pursed-lip breathing up every time I hiked up a thousand- or two-thousand-footer. Bill climbs a couple of nearby thousand-foot mountains every week during the summer, and at age seventy-nine, he hiked snowy, icy Monadnock (alt. 3,165 feet), wearing micro-spikes, a couple of times with a friend. At age sixty-seven, I still have the lung power of an eighty-year-old woman.

After eight years of the doctor looking at my cholesterol level, around 240, and saying "Diet and exercise," and me heaving another sigh of *oh-no*, I finally went to trapeze class at the circus school. The real reason I went, as well as the secondary reason I went, is a long story; so, for now, suffice it to say that the third reason I went was for exercise.

I was hooked on hanging by my knees. I just kept taking Trapeze 101. Then I realized that, in order to build some strength, I should take Circus Fit. Then they offered Flexibility 101. I have natural flexibility, so I find the flexibility class to be fun. I also attended aerial yoga for about a year, and loved using a fabric hammock suspended from the ceiling as a prop for yoga stretches. Sitting in the hammock and flipping backwards so that I was hanging upside down in the fabric felt like a really good spine stretch. And, in the four years I've been going to circus classes, I haven't lost any more height. Previously, I had already lost an inch and a quarter.

Now, because of the estrogen-inhibiting anastrozole, which will weaken my bones, the new me needs to commit to more weight-bearing exercise. I've driven past Supreme Fitness on my way into town for six years now and have never once been tempted to stop. So far, I've avoided gyms like the plague, but now the plague has struck me, so it's time to just go do the weight-bearing exercise that strengthens my bones. My friend Claire enticed me to walk into Supreme Fitness in September, and then to come to the 9:00 A.M. bone-strengthening class on Mondays and Fridays. *Cheryl, meet the weight machines.* There are about a dozen of them, each aimed at a specific muscle groups—biceps, triceps, quadriceps, calves. I trudge in on Monday and Friday mornings, but it's not so bad, really. I know many of the people there—the women with osteoporosis, the men doing their cardio rehab—all within a decade of my age. It's a good opportunity to socialize, and the music is from the sixties.

I go to the core strength class at Supreme Fitness on Tuesdays, and I've found a new Pilates class in Putney, just ten minutes away. I don't exercise to look buff or lose weight, though I am more toned and in better shape than I've ever been in my life.

When Anne turned eighty, she decided to make body maintenance a high priority and walk or kayak every day. When Nadine turned eighty-five, she started walking five miles a day. She said all her friends who didn't walk were dead.

I can understand the wisdom of *Use it or lose it.* I think of exercising as a good idea, as preventive maintenance for my high-mileage vehicle.

The new me has bought a six-month membership at the gym. I go there twice a week to work on the machines, and once or twice a week for an abs class. I've just started going to the Building Strong Bones class in Putney twice a week. I go to Pilates once a week, though I still haven't bonded with it. I'm trying to make this workout thing interesting and to fit it into my daily routine, which isn't routine at all.

Exercise every day. It's good in theory. Now to practice it.

Anastrophe

YODA IS THE master not only of The Force, but also of anastrophe—inverting the usual order of words in a sentence. "Named must your fear be before banish it you can."

Yoda also says, "Fear is the path to the dark side. Fear leads to anger. Anger leads to hate. Hate leads to suffering." Could it be true that fear of cancer is the path to the dark side? That fear of cancer leads to anger about cancer, which leads to hatred of cancer, which leads to suffering?

Receiving the diagnosis of cancer puts me in a position of anastrophe. Suddenly, the usual order of life is reversed. Suddenly, it's possible that there's not much time remaining in front of me. Suddenly, I realize that I may be at the end of my sliding scale of allotted time. All around me, friends and family are going on with their lives as if they have all the time in the world, and there's no way I can shake them awake to realize that life is precious, our time together is precious.

In his book *Being Mortal*, Atul Gawande talks about this phenomenon. Young people want to broaden their horizons and meet and spend time with new people. Meanwhile, their grandparents, knowing that not much time remains, want to spend time with those closest to them. All it takes is a shot of mortality to readjust the young person's view. If they unexpectedly lose someone close to them, they too will want to spend time with those closest to them. We sometimes can see this effect at work in the wake of disasters. After 9/11, most people wanted to stick close to home.

Now, I am in this position of anastrophe while the people around me are not. The usual order of things, the usual order of life, may be reversed. I take the drug anastrozole with the hope that *it* will reverse the usual order of cancer, as it does 85 percent of the time. Anastrozole holds the hope of reversing my current anastrophe.

Cancer is a eutrophe,[*]
perhaps an anastrophe
that feels like catastrophe.
But maybe it's just apostrophe.
Thankful I am for Buddhist philosophy.
I offer this epistrophe:[†]
Thankful I am for Buddhist philosophy.

*Train yourself to let go of
everything you fear to lose.*

— YODA

---

[*] State of nourishment (as a lake is nourished with dissolved nutrients).
[†] Repetition of a word at the end of sentences.

What I've Learned from Cancer

Surrender to life.
Say yes. Just say yes.
My mind can rest.
I don't need to worry.
No resistance required.
I'm not immortal.
I could die.
Am I ready to die?
I can get cancer.
Cancer can make itself at home in my body.
I can live with cancer.
I might die with cancer. Who knows? Who
    needs to know? Who wants to know?
Buddhism works.
Mindfulness works.
The Dharma *really* works.
The Work works.
Only two second darts. Whew!
Let it come. Let it be. Let it go. This means my
    biggest stressor. Let it loose!

So much support.

The hospital people are good people.

All the doctors are very well trained.

The nurses are kind.

The technicians are loving.

Brattleboro Memorial Hospital is easy and
     accessible.

Barbara is a really good support.

The time to set up charitable gift annuities
     is now.

Write.

Write about cancer.

I love writing my way into a new ending, a
     different angle.

My reflection books don't have to be reflection
     books.

Maybe I'm done with reflection books.

What's the cancer about? I don't know. I don't
     have to know, but I wish I knew.

Except that I'd like to know, for purposes of
     telling a story.

I have a new power of attorney and I wrote
     lengthy instructions.

It's time to do my advance directives digitally.

Maybe gardening is winding down.

I'm old. I take a prescribed medication every
     day. It's surprisingly tiny and very easy
     to swallow.

Surrendering to Life #5

ANOTHER WAY TO say "surrendering to Life" is accepting life on life's terms. Life's terms can be hard. Perhaps my term's limit is shorter than others. I want mine to be longer, but not too long. Most people I've met who are in their nineties say they are ready to go. Really, I don't have a say about the length of my lease on life. The easiest thing to do is to not have an opinion. The hardest thing for an opinionated person such as myself to do is to not have an opinion. Of course, I have an opinion about everything, but Life isn't listening to me. It's my responsibility to listen to Life. It's up to me to be in sync with Life, not the other way around.

When I signed my contract with Life, I didn't notice that it was a blank piece of paper. I really have no idea what I've agreed to. Everyone has a different contract, and it's no use comparing mine to theirs. It's no use suing Life for what I want. Life is going to win in the end.

Evelyn says that surrendering to Life takes courage and whole-heartedness. It requires courage to walk into the unknown, as she is doing with her fourth diagnosis of lymphoma. And it requires the whole-heartedness of the open heart to simply trust Life and accept things just as they are.

Nice Variations, Folks

I GO TO HITS the Spot yoga studio every Wednesday with my sweetie, Bill. The instructor, Scott, who has been teaching yoga for thirty years, was a quarterback for his high school football team, so he's a big man who does not have a typical yoga body. Due to recent knee and shoulder injuries, he often sits in a chair, giving instructions, and doing very few of the yoga poses himself. He no longer offers hands-on corrections of postures.

During every candle-lit evening class, Scott says, "It's your class. It's your body. It's your time." In other words, do your own yoga practice without concern about whether your pose looks like your neighbor's pose or that of anyone else in the class. I keep my eyes closed while doing yoga to prevent my comparing mind from snapping out any opinions about someone else's body or my own and to remain mindful of my body sensations. As we are doing a pose, he often says, "Nice variations, folks."

I sometimes do a different asana (yoga pose) from the one Scott is directing. And I have been known to lie down and do shivasana ("corpse pose"—lying supine) for the last thirty minutes of class. Sometimes this body just needs a nap instead of yoga.

We could say the same thing about life that Scott says about yoga: *It's your life. It's your body. It's your mind. It's your spirit. It's your time.*

If I am living my authentic life, my life will look different from anyone else's. Yet I've spent a lot of energy and wasted a lot of time trying to be "normal," trying to fit my round life into the square holes that "everyone else" was living—marriage, family, career, steady income. It all eluded me.

In my twenties, I wanted a boyfriend, I wanted to be coupled like "everyone else." In my thirties, I yearned for marriage and maybe children. In my forties, I met Bill, whom, twenty-seven years later, I still have not married. I tried to settle into a career, but I remained a person who switched careers every few years—human services administrator, editor and author, historian, accountant, and psychotherapist. In my fifties, I became a meditation teacher. Go figure. In my sixties, I wanted to be an active and involved grandmother like my friends. Well, I do have grandchildren (courtesy of Bill) whom I see for a few hours a year.

Trying to confine my life in the institutions of marriage, family, and career has been *completely* useless. There's only one thing left to do—give myself permission to live my authentic Cheryl life, unique in many ways, with all its diversity. It's my life. It's my time. It's my genuinely Cheryl life.

Nice variations, folks.

A Deadly Serious Opponent

BEFORE I HEARD about the two chiropractors whose breast cancer had metastasized, I had been cruising along fearlessly, amazed at the smooth, efficient, stress-free services at Brattleboro Memorial Hospital. My prognosis seemed good: the tumor was small, with clear margins and clear lymph nodes. Thanks to the millions of women who had gone before me, I felt I was on the cusp of a new generation—a generation of women who say "cancer" the way they say "urinary tract infection."

But the news about these two chiropractors brought me up short.

First of all, who was I going to see the next time my back went out of whack? I'd have to go chiropractor shopping.

But more importantly, I saw and felt that even though I had won the first three rounds, cancer is indeed a deadly serious opponent. And I mean opponent, a worthy opponent to test my strength of acceptance, positivity, and wisdom. An opponent, not an enemy, not a demon, not something to hate, not something to fear.

Rather, cancer provides me with the opportunity to

live up to it, to live through it, to live with it, to live beyond it. To come face to face with it and not flinch.

Cancer is a test. Not one to be crammed for and maybe not even one to pass and be done with. *There. That's over.* Maybe—but maybe not.

Cancer is a test to see whether I am living my practice. Cancer is a test of life. Can I surrender to Life as it is?

If cancer is a contest, I would say I won the first round, because my mind was not afraid. My body won the second round with all the good news: clear lymph nodes, clear margins, and in situ. And my genes won the third round, because I have an 85 percent chance of the cancer not recurring.

For the time being, my opponent has slunk back to his corner. I hope he's lost interest in pummeling my body, but I simply don't know.

Shall I be mired in fear of the word "cancer"? Shall I worry? Or shall I live this warm spring day when the sun is shining, birds are singing, and daffodils sway in the breeze?

Following the instructions for mindfulness, I remain calm and alert, sitting in a nonjudgmental awareness of life. Aware of the fragility of life, I feel happy for each new day.

Yes, cancer is deadly serious. But Life is deadly serious, too. Notice each moment dying to the next. Millions of cells dying, millions being born.

Today is a good day to die, but meanwhile, today, this very day, is a very good day to live—simply being present to the great life and death of Life.

Acknowledgments

T HIS BOOK AROSE from an inspiration during a ten-day meditation retreat in August 2015. The first drafts of many of these pieces were written during the five-day Sunapee Writing Retreat with Jan Frazier and Kate Gleason.

I love the women in my critiquing group—Sarah Cooper-Ellis, Sara Warner-Phillips, Melissa Hayes, and Mary Mathias—who listen deeply and prod me into new possibilities.

Thanks to Mike Fleming, the editor of this volume, who kindly pushes me to write more deeply and more thoroughly and to finally write the endings to many of these stories. Jenny Holan, proofreader extraordinaire, scrubs my manuscript clean. Oh, does that feel good! Deep appreciation to Carolyn Kasper, the award-winning designer of this book.

—*Cheryl Wilfong*
DUMMERSTON, VERMONT

cheryl.wilfong@gmail.com
cherylwilfong.com
BreastCancerMindfulness.com

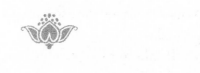

CPSIA information can be obtained
at www.ICGtesting.com
Printed in the USA
FSHW021349140619
59033FS